COMMUNITY HEALING

a transcultural model

GENEVA ENSIGN

ISBN-13: 978-0-88839-057-8 [trade edition soft-cover]
ISBN-13: 978-0-88839-119-3 [epub]
Copyright © 2018 Geneva Ensign

Library and Archives Canada Cataloguing in Publication

Ensign, Geneva, 1937-, author
Community healing : a transcultural model / Geneva
Ensign.

Includes bibliographical references and index.
Issued in print and electronic formats.
ISBN 978-0-88839-057-8 (softcover).--ISBN 978-0-88839-119-3
(EPUB)
1. Healing circles. I. Title.

BL65.M4E54 2018   615.8'52   C2018-903688-5
                                           C2018-903689-3

Printed in the USA

PRODUCTION & DESIGN: M. Lamont & D. Williams
EDITOR: D. MARTENS

In support of the truth & reconciliation movement, Hancock House and the author are pleased to commit a percentage of our sales revenues and all author royalties from this title to the Maskwacis Cultural College.

hancock

house

Published simultaneously in Canada and the United States by
HANCOCK HOUSE PUBLISHERS LTD.
19313 Zero Avenue, Surrey, B.C. Canada V3Z 9R9
(604) 538-1114   Fax (604) 538-2262

HANCOCK HOUSE PUBLISHERS
#104-4550 Birch Bay-Lynden Rd, Blaine, WA U.S.A.
98230-9436
(800) 938-1114   Fax (800) 983-2262
www.hancockhouse.com   sales@hancockhouse.com

COMMUNITY HEALING

a transcultural model

Geneva Ensign

Dedicated

to

Wilda Louis, my late co-therapist and friend,

Elder

and

founder of the

Community Wellness Program of the Samson Cree Nation

and to

all the Indigenous women, mothers and grandmothers,

who by sharing their tears and laughter

have also been

co-therapists for me

on my own journey

to Self.

To give is to receive.

TABLE OF CONTENTS

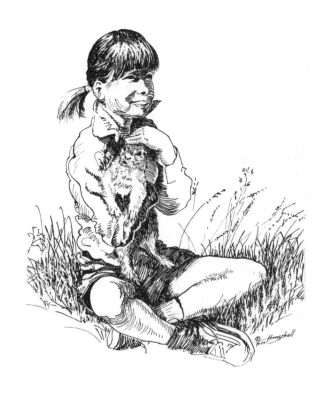

ON HEALING...

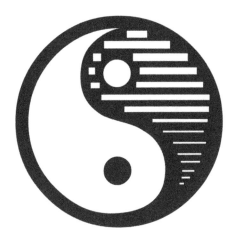

Yin-Yang: An Ancient Chinese Symbol

Healing is a process, a river, that flows back and forth from darkness to light, from pain to joy, from fear to love, if I allow it to happen.

As I heal, I swing back and forth between these opposites, but I swing less far each time if I am sincere in my effort to heal. This process underlies many cultures and is called by different names: The Warrior's Path, The Watercourse Way, The Red Road, The Path of the Heart, The Spiritual Journey.

MY SPIRIT is the guide on this journey, enabling me to become aware of my patterns, deal with my pain and break the negative cycles that often have been passed down from generation to generation.

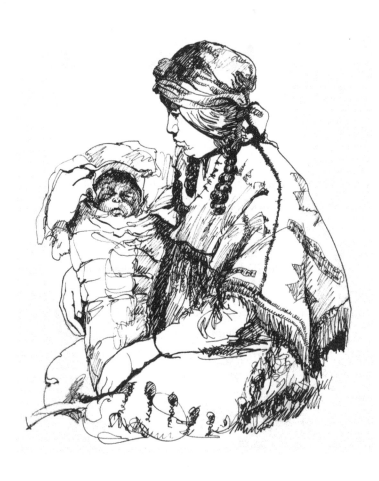

FROM THE INDIGENOUS COMMUNITY

COMMUNITY HEALING: A Transcultural Model is a compilation of the lived experience of teacher/trainer/healer Geneva Ensign's work with Indigenous groups in Canada. I met Geneva many years ago through my late aunt Wilda Louis, who was the manager of the Community Wellness Program of the Samson Cree Nation. Geneva was a facilitator, trainer and guide who first worked with the Indigenous women of my community. She was introduced to our community during the late 1970s and worked with our community until her retirement. It was during this time that I came to know her, learn from her, work with her and, eventually, grow to absolutely love her.

As I read her book, I was taken on a journey back in time; I was quickly reminded of the many Women's Healing Circles I attended in my own community, led by Geneva. The Women's Healing Circle was a small-group therapy program available for women to attend for four days away from the community. I was invited to attend the circle to begin to address and resolve the many negative emotions that I held, and I was encouraged to actively work towards healing.

I did not know too much about community development concepts or principles, but I was familiar with several psychological theories, as I was enrolled in university studies. Geneva introduced us women to psychologists such as Carl Jung and Abraham Maslow, who echoed ideas and concepts similar to Indigenous knowledge systems. Growing up, I knew that the only person I could change was myself. Geneva reinforced this idea as she stressed that personal healing leads to community healing. This idea was in line with Natural Law, a teaching I grew up knowing.

Geneva's work was always about *being with* us as Indigenous women. She never raised herself above us. As women who participated in the Healing Circles, we were all made to feel equal. She actually listened to us and she really heard us. She heard our pain, she listened to our traumatic stories, and she created a safe learning environment where she encouraged us to release our negative feelings. She called these negative emotional experiences "blocks to healing" and explained that one of the goals of the Healing Circle was to release these blocks so that positivity could return and the Spirit could flourish. She reminded us that we are all born beautiful Spirits and that we all have the potential to experience the brightness and fullness of ourselves through our deep healing work. She supported us, nurtured and respected us, and she truly loved us. We started to change.

As Indigenous women in the community, we gained strength. Eventually, we wanted to do more, and so a core group of us organized ourselves and created an annual event called the In Celebration of Women Conference to honour and celebrate the role of Indigenous women in our community. The committee members were the late Wilda Louis, Donna Potts-Johnson, Sue Buffalo, Shauna Bruno and myself. It was a successful endeavor that lasted for ten years, 1998 to 2008. Geneva guided us through this process, leading the small group facilitator training sessions.

Each of us as committee members took on a facilitation role during the conference. Little did I know that Geneva was continuing to teach and apply the community development model throughout our work.

When Geneva retired, I continued to do the work. I created several programs that I facilitated for the women in our community: one was called the *Iskwesis* (Young Girls) program and the other was called the *Omisimaw* (Eldest Sister) program. These programs were designed specifically to help women heal and to continue self-care. My university studies, along with the knowledge that I had from being raised a Maskwacis Cree, were incorporated into the training programs.

Eventually, I was inspired to obtain my doctorate degree and formulate The Omisimaw Leadership Model (four parts to the self: girl-child; sacred woman; warrior woman; wise woman). My many discussions with Geneva over the years encouraged me to write and share these teachings, and it was through her urging and support that I was able to forge ahead and obtain my doctoral degree. Throughout my own work, her teachings provided me with the foundation for understanding healing in a much deeper and broader way. Much of my work drew from the Healing Circle experiences earlier in my life.

When my Aunt Wilda passed away in May 2017, I knew that she and Geneva had claimed each other as sisters. They were similar on so many levels, particularly when it came to the topic of love. Wilda and Geneva were known to store up the hearts that they found wherever they went. Oftentimes, hearts would show up and appear in many different forms and in many different ways—glass hearts, heart-shaped rocks, heart-shaped figurines, heart-shaped rugs, heart-shaped mirrors, heart-shaped pendants, heart-shaped drawings, heart-shaped jewelry, etc. Everyone who attended Wilda's funeral was given one of these hearts. Geneva and Wilda taught that beyond skin color is Spirit, and Spirit is where love resides. This notion of love became the focal point of their work. I heard women in the community begin to say things like, "We are all Spirits having a human experience," and I knew that this awareness arose from the personal healing happening in the community.

Geneva shared many teachings that resonated with me as an Indigenous woman. In particular were the concepts of the spiral, the notion of interconnectivity, and relationality. These ideas were reminiscent of the teachings of Grandmother Spider and "all my relations" that I heard growing up, from my grandparents. The web from Grandmother Spider is the community connections among us all. These simple yet profound statements were reminders of the power that resides in us from our ancestors; they are in fact universal teachings.

In reading her book, I did not realize that Geneva was given opportunities to receive a traditional name. As the universe would unfold in our journey together, a name was given to me to give to her a few days after my aunt's funeral. In our discussion about her work, I told Geneva that I saw her as a Rainbow Ribbon Carrier Woman, and so it is with great pride that I introduce her to you all as such.

In this time of reconciliation between and amongst Indigenous and non-Indigenous peoples, there is a doorway opening to allow for love and Spirit to grow. It this through this type of seminal work that others can learn how to facilitate such a process so that humanity may all benefit. This was the prophecy of our Indigenous people. And it shall be. Transcultural community healing is being called for, and Rainbow Ribbon Carrier Woman lays out a pathway for others to follow.

Claudine Louis, B.A., B.Ed., M.Ed., Ph.D.
President, Maskwacis Cultural College
Maskwacis, Alberta
June 2017

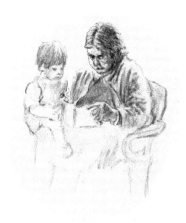

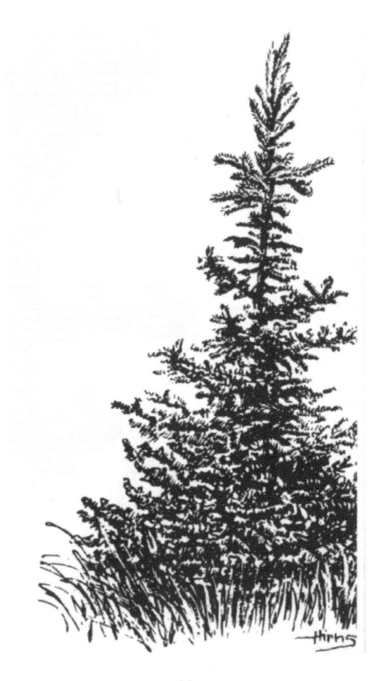

FROM
THE NON-INDIGENOUS
COMMUNITY

IT IS AN honour and a pleasure to write a foreword to Geneva Ensign's new book, *Community Healing: A Transcultural Model*. Geneva distills her decades of experience and wisdom into a powerful, practical and visionary model. It is, through and through, a strengths-based book about healing the wounds that beset individuals, families and communities.

The book begins by taking us on a historical journey through the evolution of holistic approaches to education and training for personal, professional and community development. Many of us who joined community colleges, including Grant MacEwan Community College, as instructors in the early '70s were captivated by the ideas of experiential and holistic education. Alberta, in particular, was going through a time of dramatic increase in services but also a critical shortage of trained professionals. As educators, we were captured by the possibilities of adapting more traditional programs and educational approaches in order to reach those who might not otherwise have access to personal and career education.

Geneva was an important innovator and a role model for others in the development and delivery of workshop-based outreach programming in Indigenous communities. Her work unlocked a treasure chest of possibilities. I particularly recall the exciting curriculum on "community" that she developed with students in a weeklong workshop on the banks of the Yukon River. She worked from the heart then, and still does. She truly believed that students and teachers could learn together, and still does.

Though she is deeply embedded as an "informed outsider" in knowledge and respect for Indigenous people and cultural traditions, Geneva wisely avoids the trap of writing a recipe book for Indigenous education. In choosing, rather, to build on a transcultural model, and to offer the reader a collection of holistic approaches, she broadens the relevance of her ideas for expanded contemporary training and development. She does not succumb to the temptation to say we are all alike in the human family, leading to a one-size-fits-all approach to education. Rather, we should work with humility to transcend cultural boundaries and to discover the human qualities and aspirations we do share.

This is all the more important in an era of Reconciliation, an era of increasing Indigenous self-determination in education and service delivery, and an era of increasing cultural diversity in the Canadian population generally. We are, in my estimation, in the midst of a managerial era in education and service delivery, an era that demands more information, more results and an objective analysis of issues—but so often dismisses the importance of relationship, community, nature, and a focus on the whole person. I recommend Geneva's book as an antidote. As she says, "There is a new dance in town." Or can be.

Duane Massing, RSW, PhD
Professor Emeritus (Social Work)
MacEwan University
June 2017

PREFACE

THE TRANSCULTURAL MODEL for Community Healing outlined here grew organically out of my forty-plus years of personal and professional involvement in human relations training and counselling in Indigenous and non-Indigenous communities and organizations. This involvement ranged from community level workshops, program development and teaching in the outreach program of a community college, and organization planning for community and government agencies as well as individual and group psychotherapy.

Armed with a B.Ed. and an M.A. in community development, I, a non-Indigenous person, began my career in Indigenous communities while one of five partners in Co-West Associates, a small social planning and research company in Edmonton, Alberta. We were under contract with Grant MacEwan Community College (now MacEwan University) to develop and facilitate community development training modules that would be delivered on Indigenous reserves in Alberta and Yukon.

These modules were part of an outreach program that would enable Indigenous persons employed as paraprofessional helpers on the reserves to begin a two-year program that would end in a Social Services Worker (later Social Work) diploma. For the second year of the program, students would enroll at Grant MacEwan in Edmonton. It was hoped that from there they could transfer to a BSW program at Calgary or other schools of social work. This visionary program was one of the first outreach programs offered by an accredited college in Alberta. It was an exciting and innovative idea for that time in the mid-'70s.

Over the next few years, I was hired to develop and facilitate additional human relations training workshops, i.e., decision-making, organizational development, interpersonal communication, group dynamics and personal awareness. I discovered quickly that working on the reserve was vastly different from teaching at a community college in an urban setting. It did not take long for me, and my colleagues, to discover that the traditional lecture method was not effective, that curriculum and teaching methods designed for urban areas and university-oriented educational programs did not work well in an Indigenous community. As we struggled to find new ways of teaching, I discovered that I was only just beginning my own learning process.

We needed to develop new approaches to teaching and learning, and this required a new mindset. As we began to experiment with various experiential learning exercises to teach the principles and practice of community development, the students themselves told us what worked and what did not. We were in a new-to-us educational environment, one of experiential learning, where each person in the workshops, including ourselves, was both teacher and learner.

In addition, I was going through a period of my own personal growth and change, often spurred by challenges in the individual and community counselling in which I was involved. I began to attend as many training programs as I could. I enrolled in a variety of therapies, i.e., gestalt, transactional analysis, dream work, relaxation and stress reduction, psychodrama and the Institute for Intensive Therapy. I also became a Registered Social Worker and was accepted as a full member in the Canadian Group Psychotherapy Association. The dual role, composed of my own personal growth and the facilitation of personal growth and healing for Indigenous social workers in training, was the crucible in which this grassroots training model for community healing emerged.

For a non-Indigenous woman to work in Indigenous communities involves—and always has—a delicate balance. During the early 1970s many helpers would attempt to adopt the local culture in order to be accepted in the community. Conversely, other non-Indigenous helpers would revert to being an authority figure and instruct via a traditional textbook model. I learned by experience that it was okay for me to come as myself, a non-Indigenous person with ideas to share and open to the workshop participants, who also had life experiences and wisdom to share. When we looked across the cultural divide at this human level, we discovered the commonalities that united us rather than the differences that divided.

Over the span of my career, I have facilitated many variations of human relations workshops, not only for Indigenous organizations and communities, but in non-Indigenous settings as well. In this process, I have learned that *the fundamental principles and practices of healing are transcultural;* they can be applied to any group or community that is willing to undergo a healing process. Transcultural is defined here as the concepts and beliefs that underlie and transcend cultural boundaries, encompassing what it means *to be a member of the human family*. For the purposes of this book, I want to focus on how this transcultural model can be applied in Indigenous communities.

I usually avoid the use of *should,* whether working with an individual or with a community. *Should* is a prescription for action, informing another of what they ought to do, rather than encouraging them to make their own self-responsible choices. However, some issues are so important that I do use *should* to highlight these. Similarly, I use the word *wholistic,* rather than the more proper *holistic,* to underscore the meaning of being complete, whole, well. The words *healing circles* and *workshops* are used interchangeably as well.

When I first began my career in the 1970s, the words Native and Indian were acceptable usages, i.e., Native Counselling Services of Alberta and Indian Affairs. I still slip up sometimes, but I am choosing to use the term Indigenous out of respect for the changes that have occurred over the years. I have been told that many Indigenous people prefer it because it means "arising naturally from a region or a country." Arising naturally is a beautiful concept, implying health, wholeness and connectedness with the world around.

Admittedly, my work in Indigenous communities spans a long time frame; much has changed in those years. However, much stays the same. The nature of what it means to belong to the human family remains unchanged.

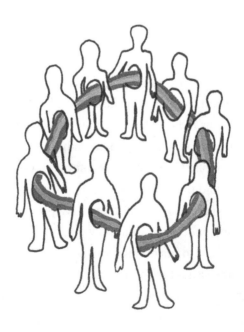

ACKNOWLEDGMENTS

A CAREER OF FORTY-PLUS years leaves a cohort of many friends, family, colleagues and employers without whom my career, and therefore this book, would have never happened. I start first with Co-West Associates, an Edmonton-based research and training group of which I was one of five associates.

Native Counselling Services of Alberta was the first Indigenous group to contract with me personally to facilitate workshops. To Chester Cunningham, founder and president, Doug Heckbert, training coordinator, to Amanda Golosky, co-facilitator of personal awareness workshops, and to Elder Wilton Goodstriker for his words of wisdom, I will be forever grateful.

The Social Work Department of Grant MacEwan College, now a university, hired Co-West Associates to develop and facilitate the first community development learning modules for their innovative long-distance Social Work Training Program on Alberta reserves. Dr. Duane Massing was especially helpful and encouraging in my group work, allowing me to develop new experiential learning modules, as requested by the Indigenous communities.

Sylvester Jack, former chief of the Atlin Indian Band, and his daughter, Louise Gordon, the band manager, spearheaded a community wellness process. Our work with them was instrumental in our formulating new and exciting ways to work in communities. Many changes have taken place since then and Louise is now chief/spokesperson for the band and the co-author of Chapter 7, "Community Visioning: The Case of Taku River Tlingit First Nation."

A huge debt of gratitude goes to the late Wilda Louis, founder and director of the Community Wellness Program, Samson Band, Maskwacis, Alberta. She contracted with me to conduct residential Women's Therapy Groups as five-day intensive workshops. Over the years, she became my co-therapist, and, after my retirement in 2005, she continued to conduct the therapy groups on her own. She was seen as an Elder, and we came to claim each other as sisters.

More recently, as I prepare this book for publication, I have a different group of people to thank, namely, the Westbank Writers' Group and Blair Jean, co-facilitator and author of *Clearwater Memoirs*. They all generously shared their time, advice and encouragement for this project. Also, thank you, Crystal Anne Williams, for turning my rough sketches into computer graphics. Norma Hill, Marie Waddell, Ike and Millie Glick, Gail Cowie, each with a sharp eye and editing pencil, offered crucial suggestions and corrections. My publishers deserve credit, Myles Lamont for endless patience with my many questions and David Hancock for encouraging me to "go further."

At a personal level, I am aware that my children often had no choice about sharing their mother with her career. It was not always easy for them, but I am eternally grateful to Greg, Geri and Grant for their love and understanding. Lastly, acknowledgment goes to my late husband, colleague and dear friend, Bob Langin. We journeyed many miles together, both personally and professionally. He was a great listener, sounding board and inspiration throughout my entire career.

Thank you all.

ENDORSEMENTS

"Community Healing: A Transcultural Model outlines a pathway to healing for individuals and communities, reminding us all that the rediscovery of Spirit provides the motivation and direction for our healing journeys. The Model is based on the belief that as individuals within a community heal, so does the community.

I wholeheartedly endorse this book as a valuable resource in implementing our vision for healing and reconciliation."

**-- Dr. Wilton Littlechild, IPC
Grand Chief
Treaty Six Confederacy**

"Community Healing A Transcultural Model by Geneva Ensign expertly captures the basic understanding that must be comprehended before one can teach, train or profess to heal oneself or a community. It is a teaching tool that I highly recommend. Being an Aboriginal leader for many years and growing up on the reserve surrounded by the traditional teachings of my Stemtemma (Grandmother), I understand our culture and its importance. To be ready for the future, we must understand the past. The compilation of stories and experiences presented in this book gives a wholesome insight as to what we, as Indigenous People, are all about.

I highly recommend and endorse Geneva's book."

**-- Robert Louie
Former Chief of Westbank First Nation
LL.B, OC, Hon. Dr. LL.B**

"It is my pleasure to personally endorse the Community Healing: A Transcultural Model. Our community has been greatly impacted by the effects of the Residential School and have been taking the initiative to support the Truth and Reconciliation recommendations.

Thank you for the opportunity to host and offer our support."

-- Chief Vern Saddleback
Samson Cree Nation

"I fully endorse The Community Healing: A Transcultural Model as a significant framework that will enhance our Maskwacis community towards healing. The journey as an individual alone is much harder than the community as a whole. This holistic model provides us with the aspiration to heal generations to come."

-- Jerry Saddleback
MCC Elder
Maskwacis Cultural College

PART ONE

OUTLINING AN ALTERNATIVE MODEL FOR COMMUNITY HEALING

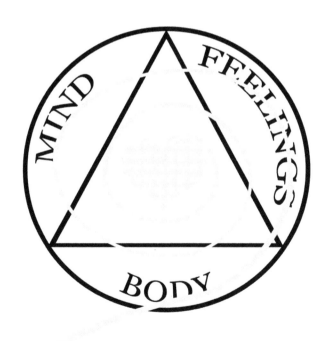

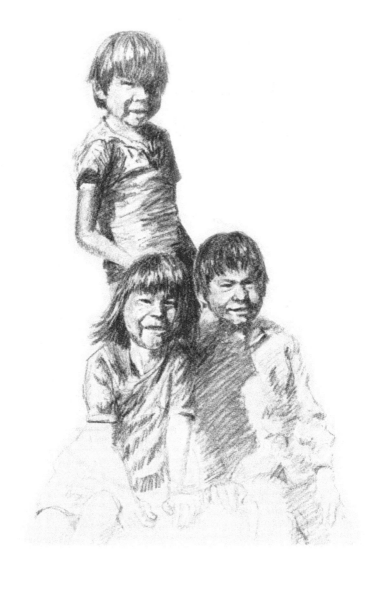

CHAPTER 1

COMMUNITY HEALING: A TRANSCULTURAL MODEL

"If you can't draw a picture, you don't understand it."

THE MODEL, AS APPLIED TO INDIGENOUS COMMUNITIES

THE NEED FOR the healing of Indigenous communities has long been recognized. Since the beginning of European contact, Indigenous communities in Canada have been torn between two (at least) very different worlds, between conflicting value systems and between very different cultural ways of being in the world. As the non-Indigenous culture became more and more dominant, Indigenous communities had less and less control over fundamental decision-making processes for their people and for their communities. This loss of control resulted in a breakdown in traditional ways, which brought about many personal and social problems.

Educational and training programs designed by the dominant culture tended to further increase the gulf between the two ways of being. The full story of the disastrous effect of residential schools on individuals and communities is still being told, as is the effect on communities of social welfare programs that were designed to help. Instead, the programs often further increased dependency and alienation. This was graphically described by Peter Erasmus, an Alberta Metis who was born and raised in northern Alberta, in a book, *Practical Framework for Community Liaison Work.*

> *My grandmother had a self-sufficient way of life. She had a small, manageable farm, lived off the land, went to church, worked hard and raised her children—and her grandchildren...*
>
> *Then ... officials came from an urban setting; they did not understand the life and the values of the people out here. I believe that the communities and government are still dealing with the effects of how the "welfare" was brought to our area...*
>
> *In one family, money was very, very scarce, but they had three cows and a team of horses. They heard that other people in the area were getting something called "social assistance." They inquired about it. The welfare officials asked them what they had. They were told, "If you get rid of all that, you will qualify." So they got rid of their cows and the team.*
>
> *Almost overnight, many of the people said, "Why not? If we can get it for nothing, why should we work for it?" That started a mentality that has grown ... after a while, the children and the grandchildren have never known another way.*
>
> – Erasmus, 1991, p. 3.

In the 1960s, community development programs were initiated in Alberta, the tacit goal of which was to transfer power from government back to the Indigenous communities so that they could take charge of their own destinies. Community developers were hired to work with communities to bring this transformation about, the purpose of which was to empower communities through a self-help philosophy.

The story of community development in Alberta is an interesting one. Development meant different things to different people—economic development, human resource development, the provision of services, educational programs and community programs *to get people organized* in order to function more effectively—usually according to a government-developed plan. All programs were primarily aimed at getting individuals and communities off welfare and helping them to become self-sufficient.

The results were a mixed bag: massive problems continued on reserves despite, and often because of, government attempts. When Indigenous people did voice their concerns and make their needs and wants known, government officials were alarmed. Community development programs were supposed to result in costing the government less money, not more. Subsequently, the government's community development programs were abandoned or absorbed into other government departments; *community development* became a taboo phrase, and workers were fired or were assigned to other helping roles in Indigenous communities. Other attempts to address Indigenous issues ensued. Universities, community colleges and private training companies developed many different programs *to solve the Indian problem*, as seen through the eyes of the non-Indigenous community.

Now, many years later, Indigenous community members are taking back the role of helper. All over Canada, Indigenous communities are in various stages of settling their land claims, are designing their own governing and business systems, and are actively involved in issues of community reorganization and healing. However, major problems still exist. Some helpers are working almost night and day on reserves to intervene in what seems like a chronic cycle of abuse, addictions of various kinds, and suicide. We only have to look to the attempts to help the following communities to understand the enormity of the challenge as well as to listen thoughtfully and empathetically to the dehumanizing stories of abuse in residential schools experienced by their residents: Davis Inlet in Newfoundland and Labrador, Kashechewan in Northern Ontario, Pimicikamak in Manitoba, or La Loche of Saskatchewan.

Unanswered questions abound. As Indigenous people assume responsibility for their own governing and for their social and educational systems, will they adapt the former policies and programs or develop a truly new Indigenous system? If so, upon whose values and traditions will it be based? As Indigenous people advocate for their rightful place in the wider society, how will a melding of the old and new take place? On whose terms? The questions and dilemmas seem endless to decision-makers and planners in Indigenous communities and in government.

THE CRUCIAL QUESTION

I believe the most crucial question is: How can community development take place when so many community members need personal healing? This often overlooked truth was identified when the participants in one of the community development training modules said to me, "What we are learning in this community development workshop is important and valuable to us as community helpers, but how can we truly help our clients when our own lives are falling apart? We need a chance to heal ourselves before we can really help our clients." Community helpers and healers are often so busy dealing with crises—their own as well as their clients'—that they haven't had time to wonder about the basic underlying issue, as defined in a story titled, "Where Are the Bodies Coming From?"

The story is about a village that was located beside a river. One day, the inhabitants of the village noticed, to their surprise and horror, that there were people floating downstream. Some were lifeless bodies; others, barely alive, were clinging desperately to logs. Being kind-hearted people, the villagers rushed out into the river and rescued them. They carried the living into their homes and gave them food and loving care. They buried those who had drowned.

In a few days' time, more bodies floated down the river, clinging to logs and deadfalls. Again, the villagers waded into the river, bringing them into their homes to care for them. After a few days' time, more were seen floating downstream, exhausted, and clinging to whatever would keep them afloat. Again, the people of the village went out, rescued them and brought them into their village. Weeks went by.

There were now many "river people" in the village, all needing housing, food and care. The village houses were filled to overflowing; the cemetery, too, was overcrowded. Some villagers were assigned to full-time river rescue work; others were assigned to full-time house building; other members of the community were assigned to full-time care for the ever-increasing number of bodies.

Years went by. And the bodies kept coming. Since the village was small, the extra demand on personal and village resources put the villagers under severe strain.

They became exhausted, then angry. They no longer treated the river people with love and care. They no longer treated each other with love. They could not even care for themselves and their families. They were so busy and so tired. Soon, they no longer cared at all—about anything. Everything appeared hopeless.

One day, a child of the village was standing beside the river. He looked upstream; yet more bodies came floating into view. With the clarity of vision that children often have, he quietly asked, "Where are all the bodies coming from?" No one had asked that question before; no one had thought to go upstream to find the "source" of the crisis that was overwhelming the village. In fact, in the midst of the survival efforts, they had not even wondered about it …

– Anonymous

I heard a version of the above story for the first time while living and working in Yukon. As with most stories and fables, its origin has been lost in its telling and retelling. However, the point is very clear: If you don't know what is broken, how can you know what to fix?

Previously, it was mostly the non-Indigenous community who tried to identify and fix what they called *The Indian Problem*. Today, more and more Indigenous voices are speaking up and identifying what's wrong and what's been wrong for a very long time. The so-called *Indian Problem* started with a colonial way of being governed. The list of inhumane practices goes on and on: the shame and horror of what happened to children in residential schools, the outlawing of Indigenous spiritual practices, the practice of herding people into reserves that were governed by Indian agents and giving them new names or numbers to replace their Indigenous names.

It is easy to become discouraged when attempting to develop plans to deal with overwhelming community problems—cultural, social, political, educational, economic and organizational. Where does one start? In the attempt to fix what was wrong, many helpers and communities have settled for obvious, but surface, solutions: more money, more housing units, more indoor plumbing, even more social workers, psychologists and nurses. There is a great temptation to opt for obvious solutions to *deal with the bodies.*

THE NEED TO RE-ESTABLISH PERSONAL POWER

However, the issue could be examined in a different, deeper light. Over years and years of colonial contact with the white world, Indigenous individuals and communities became subjugated to the dominant culture. In this process, they lost their *power.* Personal power can be defined as self-worth, self-love, personal dignity and the ability to make the decisions that shape one's life and one's world. Being dominated, which results in feelings of powerlessness, leads to anger. This anger is often turned inward toward oneself, one's family or one's community. Hence, the multitude of social issues that bedevil efforts for change. When anger does not change the situation and only makes it worse, hopelessness and apathy take over. There is no more Spirit left, just bleak hopelessness that leads to sickness, abuse, murder and suicide.

Indigenous communities cannot effectively deal with the community issues unless personal power, self-worth and self-determination are re-established. Otherwise, no matter how much money and how many resources and programs are poured into a community, there still is no foundation on which to move forward. It is time for deep introspection in an attempt to understand the underlying dynamics of Indigenous communities that are in crisis and to develop programs that will, in fact, facilitate individual and community healing.

This deep introspection has begun, especially illustrated by the Truth and Reconciliation Commission. These Canada-wide hearings, coupled with the investigation into Missing and Murdered Indigenous Women, have provided powerful legitimization for the need that Indigenous persons have to tell their stories, talk about their pain *and to be heard*. These commissions have heightened society's awareness of the need for healing in the Indigenous community and in the non-Indigenous community as well. The time is right; the tide is beginning to change. I would like to add my thoughts and dreams toward a collective vision of what could possibly staunch the flow of bodies down the river.

My professional and personal experiences in Indigenous communities over the years provided me with a wonderful opportunity to observe the dynamics between individuals within a community and between communities and outside authorities. I would like to present some very basic concepts, stripped to their essence, in an attempt to examine where the *bodies* are coming from. I will also present some ideas on what can be done to facilitate healing for individuals and communities.

Years ago, an Indigenous woman, an Elder, challenged me, "You white people! You talk a lot without understanding. If you can't draw a picture, you don't understand!" Her wise challenge motivated me to try to delve below the surface issues to capture the underlying concepts and principles—the simple truths that underlie sometimes very complicated theories. Interestingly enough, she was in agreement with Einstein when he said, "If you can't explain it simply, you don't understand it well enough." Often, in workshops, simple word pictures and images would emerge that encapsulated the issues we were dealing with, illustrating that, in essence, healing is a very basic and natural human process, truly transpersonal and transcultural. The simple but profound illustrations that accompany the text came from these workshops, as the participants and I struggled to really understand the personal, interpersonal and community issues. The images helped to give form and substance to intangible truths about human nature and healing.

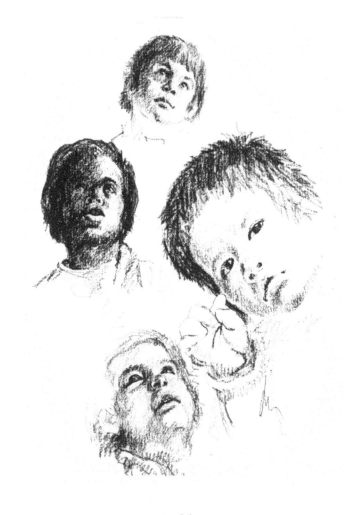

CHAPTER 2

ON COMMUNITY

"Community=an invisible web
of self-made bonds between people."

COMMUNITY: WHAT IS IT?

COMMUNITY IS A common word, one that we all use easily, but we seldom stop to ponder what a community *really* is. In simplistic terms, a community is obviously a physical place with houses, schools, stores, sewers, a system of economics, and some type of local governance, with agencies for various service delivery programs.

Community development programs have traditionally focused on these tangible aspects of community. Yet, underneath the tangible aspects, there is an invisible community. It could be described as a collection of individuals plus *something more*. The *something more* comprises extensive, but invisible, *webs* of shared language, values, beliefs, traditions, symbols and emotions, both positive and negative ones. This invisible community exerts a powerful influence on, and structures, the visible one.

For centuries, within the structure of these invisible webs, individuals in communities have set their own rules and governed themselves according to their commonalities, both formally and

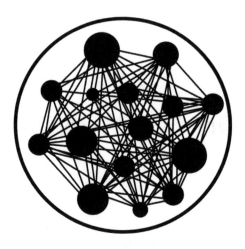

Figure 1 "Invisible Community Webs"

informally. The totality of these webs, created over time, comprises a way of being and doing that *is* culture.

It was these felt connections between people, the webs, that community development workers largely ignored or failed to see. It is important to understand these fundamental and seemingly simple dynamics when attempting to design any programs meant for community development and/or community healing.

At its basic level, the relationship between an individual and the community is an interactive and very powerful two-way socialization process. It works something like this: an individual is born not only into their family, but also into the complicated web of relationships that make up the community. This new community member is shaped and molded by these powerful visible and invisible webs. This process is like the air one breathes; one is not conscious of being taught specific ways of being and doing. It is just the way it is—whether or not those ways of being and doing are positive or negative for the individual's wellbeing, or the community's.

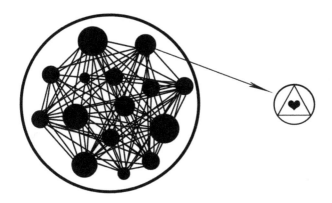

Figure 2 "Community Shaping the Individual"

Above is a diagram depicting the community's webs, exerting their power to socialize a new member into the community's ways.

However, the individual is not just a blank slate open to being molded and shaped by the community; each individual has the ability, the power, to react to the forces of socialization. By so doing, the individual also helps to mold and reshape the community, knowingly or unknowingly, positively or negatively.

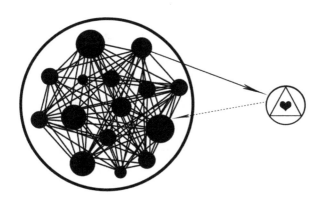

Figure 3 "The Individual Reacting and Shaping Community"

This is a dynamic, ever-changing, relationship—that of the individual and the community. Of course, the community is made up of many individuals in various combinations: one-on-one relationships, family groups, extended family groups or clans, interest groups, and organizations, formal and informal. Again, simply put, in ever-widening circles, these invisible and dynamic webs are the *building blocks* of community and of the larger society.

Community development practice is based on the fundamental belief that within each individual lies the wisdom and potential for healthy and natural growth and change. In fact, within each person lies a directional force, an innate pull, toward growth.

When individuals choose the path of healing, all the invisible webs of which they are a part are directly affected. Relationships are automatically affected, thereby necessitating some type of reaction. When a part of the whole (an individual) changes, the whole (the community) has changed as well. This is inevitable. The deeper and more profound the changes in the individual, the more profound are the changes in the wider community. This is a powerful dynamic.

When independent, strong people work together in the community for the good of the whole, healthy, strong bonds are forged at every level. Individuals then are operating from their personal power, power being the ability to make things happen. Personal power is having the ability to be in charge of oneself and having the inner and outer resources to make decisions that provide not only for survival but also for growth and development of the individual.

In other words, personal power means the ability to be independent and yet able to work together with other community members for the good of the whole. This is the definition of interdependence. A community is strongest when its ways of being and doing are created and sustained by the community members working together. Robert Nisbet, in his book, *Quest for Community*, calls these self-made webs "social authority."

A workshop early in my career graphically taught me the difference between self-made webs and ways of doing things imposed from outside the community. My partner and I were facilitating a community development workshop for the leaders of an Indigenous community; our task for one session was to present a blueprint within which the community leaders could analyze their community's decision-making process. This blueprint was a well-known one called the Force Field Analysis. It was a very popular model in human relations training at the time.

Our task was to teach the workshop participants this process, having them list the community's issues, identify and analyze various solutions, set priorities and timelines, and allocate specific jobs. Overall, this was a pretty comprehensive, but non-Indigenous, model for community planning. However, the participants resisted working with the Force Field Analysis, saying that their community had its own model for planning, that they did not need "ours"!

Fortunately, we knew enough not to insist on following the pre-set community college curriculum. Instead, we asked them to share with us their decision-making model. A word picture emerged that beautifully illustrated how they perceived the relationship between social authority and externally imposed interventions into their community. They said:

When you go outside in the early morning and the sun is shining on the dewy blades of grass, you can see fine, almost invisible, webs. Those webs are just like our connection with each other in our community. It is by these webs that decisions are made, communicated to each other and events get organized. It works for us.

Then a person from government comes along to help us and steps in the middle of our web with his big feet. He doesn't even realize what he has just done. Then he asks, "Why don't you guys get organized!"

Understanding the nature of these very basic relationships—that of the individual and community and of the community and outside authorities—is fundamental to the Transcultural Healing Model.

HOW COMMUNITIES BECOME "UNWELL"

The foregoing description is an ideal picture; the reality is different. When a community exists in the midst of a dominant society whose ways of being are contrary to the smaller community, and when this dominant society has power over the community, the very webs that hold a community together are slowly eroded.

Many books have been written about the effects of colonialism on Indigenous communities. Being made wards of the state, being given numbers instead of names, being removed from their traditional lands, being forcibly placed in abusive residential schools and not being allowed to speak their language are just some examples of colonial practices. In June 2016, CBC News reported that almost half of non-Indigenous people who were polled believed that residential schools were responsible for the problems facing communities.

Certainly, almost 100 percent of the Indigenous people in Canada also ascribe blame to the government, its policies, and the colonial mentality that has existed since first contact—and still does. Suffice it to say, every aspect of community was, and still is, dealing with a powerfully negative impact, tragic results passed down from generation to generation. Today it is being called lateral violence.

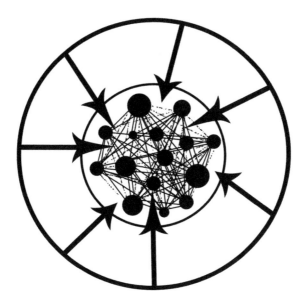

Figure 4 "Community Being Impacted By Outside Forces"

When a community's ways of being are undermined, individuals within that community begin to feel lost and alienated from themselves and from one another. People lose their sense of who they are; they lose their independence, their autonomy and their ability to make the decisions necessary for the continuation of their way of being. At a personal and community level, this *is* powerlessness at its most basic. Powerlessness always breeds negative feelings: worry, frustration, anxiety, anger, rage, fear, and self-hatred—and, therefore, hatred of others. When individuals are powerless to confront an outside authority, they tend to turn their hurt and anger against themselves, their own family, friends and community members. When hope for change is gone, individuals become increasingly despairing and, eventually, apathetic or violent.

It is a psychological truth that feelings of low self-esteem and self-hatred are turned either inward or outward, depending on the personality of the individual—inward to self or outward to family and fellow community members, or both. This is a vicious cycle that spirals ever downward, destroying from within the very webs that a person and a community need for their survival. In essence, most social problems can be explained by hatred of oneself turned inward or outward. The individual has become their own enemy.

Figure 5 shows how negative feelings and self-hatred are played out in progressively more destructive ways. When the community's self-ruling and self-regulating ways of being begin to crumble, a reinforcing cycle of disintegration has been set in motion. A power vacuum has been created. It is then that additional outside authorities step in, sometimes with good intentions, but unfortunately often with intentions that primarily suit their own agenda—to rescue, to educate, to convert, to conquer or to colonize.

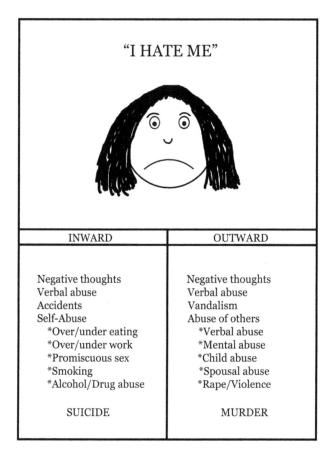

"I HATE ME"

INWARD	OUTWARD
Negative thoughts	Negative thoughts
Verbal abuse	Verbal abuse
Accidents	Vandalism
Self-Abuse	Abuse of others
*Over/under eating	*Verbal abuse
*Over/under work	*Mental abuse
*Promiscuous sex	*Child abuse
*Smoking	*Spousal abuse
*Alcohol/Drug abuse	*Rape/Violence
SUICIDE	MURDER

Figure 5 "Self-Hatred Turned Inward, Outward"

The relationship between a community and an outside authority is a dynamic, interactive and usually destructive force because the ability to choose, to be self-governing, is fundamental to ongoing maintenance of one's way of being. When decisions are made for a community, or an individual, that they could or should make for themselves, they are being conditioned to become dependent rather than independent. The more decisions an outside authority makes for the community, the more control it assumes over that community, the more the invisible webs disintegrate, little by little. The more dependent the community becomes, the larger and stronger the outside authority grows. It is a subtle, debilitating dynamic, usually in the name of helping.

The late Peter Erasmus described eloquently the disintegration of his Metis grandparents' way of life when the government promised community members welfare if they would quit their traditional ways of providing for themselves—growing gardens, hunting, fishing and trapping. In just over a generation, welfare became a way of life for a formerly independent community.

Community disintegration sometimes is so total that people in positions to implement community development or community healing programs often are confused and overwhelmed, wondering where to begin. To attempt to address the broken webs of individuals and of communities with the usual solutions—better houses, schools, sewers or even more money—is to fail to address the root causes of the disintegration. However, that is not to belittle the desperate needs of people in communities for these amenities.

HOW COMMUNITIES BECOME WELL AGAIN

Community Development: A Framework

Community development is a *process* in which community members come together to work on issues held in common. It is a way of facilitating people to become involved in defining and solving their own issues. These programs were not designed to work on psychological or spiritual issues of the individuals in community but on broader communal issues. Yet, the underlying philosophy of community development does provide a *framework* within which community healing can take place.

In 1970, Arthur Dunham developed a list of principles and practices that he published under the title "The Nature and Characteristics of Community Development." These principles and the ensuing ways of working in a community are profound and, if understood and implemented, will begin a process of change. They can provide an overall blueprint for subsequent community healing programs.

COMMUNITY PLANNING PRINCIPLES

PRINCIPLES:

▶ Every person in a community is valuable and *has inherent worth and dignity.*

▶ *Self-determination* is a basic right and responsibility of individuals and groups, meaning the ability to make decisions individually and with others for the good of the group.

▶ Within each person are *the desire and the ability* to learn, grow and develop.

▶ Growth implies *positive development* in all aspects of one's self: Body, Mind, Feelings, and Spirit.

▶ Each individual has a unique contribution to make to the *life* of a community.

▶ Community change *happens* as individuals within it grow and change.

THEREFORE, COMMUNITY PLANNING WILL:

▶ Be concerned with the overall well-being of all community members

- ▶ Be concerned with facilitating growth by deliberate, conscious action and planning

- ▶ Integrate and use knowledge and expertise from all disciplines

- ▶ Work with community people in various combinations: Individuals, one-to-one, small groups, inter-group and the community as a whole

- ▶ Be based in self-help and self-responsibility

- ▶ Be based in participation, involvement and cooperative action

- ▶ Work with self and/or community identified issues, not pre-determined agendas

- ▶ Use conscious decision-making or general agreement, not majority win

- ▶ Emphasize process (people participation and cooperation) over a pre-determined result

- ▶ Be long-term, not a crash program

– Adapted from Dunham, 1970, 172-173.

In the late 1970s, Grant MacEwan Community College in Edmonton, Alberta, initiated an innovative outreach program designed to provide first year social work training to Indigenous people in their own community. The community development segments of this social work program were designed as experiential workshops in which participants would examine their own community, using the above principles and practices, a *learning by doing* approach.

Following each workshop, participants were asked to evaluate the workshop and assess its applicability to their community work. Participants consistently rated the workshops as being extremely helpful, and they reported that they now had some new ways of working and new awarenesses with which to facilitate community development.

Going Deeper: Dealing with Personal Problems

However, workshop participants returning for subsequent community development modules said that something was still missing, even though the workshops were helping them work with their communities more effectively. Though they were the leaders in their communities, they said that their personal lives and their relationships were falling apart. Wondering how they could help others when they could not even help themselves, they requested some sessions that would help them understand and deal with their personal problems. Since self-identified need is one of the basic practices of community development, the social work department at Grant MacEwan added a personal development segment to the curriculum.

Interesting things began to happen. Not only did individuals work on themselves, but strong bonds began to be forged between group members. Relationships between participants began to heal. As they experienced new ways of being with each other, they began to put these in practice back home with their families and in their jobs.

The community leaders involved in these workshops had provided their own answer to the question of how they could begin a healing process for their community. Their answer, of course, was that communities needed to begin with a community development process that truly deals with the *core* of the problem; that individuals within a community need to heal before they can be effective helpers and leaders. In this way, community development had added a new level, that of personal healing at a community level.

Going Even Deeper: Indigenous Elders

The need to address the brokenness of individuals and communities was affirmed years ago by Wilton Goodstriker, Elder and spiritual leader from the Kainai Reserve in southern Alberta. In 1988, he spoke at the annual general meeting of Native Counselling Services for their province-wide staff and affiliated agencies. His topic was "Spirituality and Community Healing."

He said that his Boss, the Creator, had given him a purpose. That purpose was to take care of his body and his Spirit. "This," he said, "is also the job of all people in the human family." He thought that Indigenous communities had become unhealthy because the people had lost their freedom. He said that his

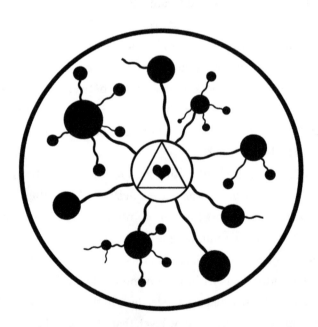

*Figure 6 "As Individuals Heal, the
Community's Webs Do Also"*

forefathers had known how to be free and to control their Spirits, but that now the people had allowed their bodies and Spirits to be controlled. He believed that individuals and communities became lost and failed without this vital, life-giving connection to Spirit.

He went on to say, "We doubt ourselves because we don't control ourselves. We want to be someone else, someone like the white man. Why can't we take charge of our Spirits again and be our own selves? Culture is still here; we're the ones who have become lost."

In essence, he was saying that Spirit is still alive and well somewhere deep within each individual, no matter how lost or broken. Rediscovery of this Spirit, or Inner Self, lies at the core of individual and community healing. Rediscovery of the Inner Self begins a process of reintegrating an individual's personal power and, when an individual makes changes, these changes affect their web of relationships.

He ended his presentation by saying that Spirit had prophesied a long time ago that communities would return to *the Good*. He said that all people are gifted differently, but that all gifts point to *the oneness of all*. He said that we are *all* here in the world to be a part of *the One*, including Mother Earth. He continued to counsel that it is important to heal, and that to heal is to be helpful to one another and to search within oneself for the lost Spirit. "That's healing," he said, "but change and healing have a price, that of pain and separation from the old negative ways."

He concluded his remarks by saying that he is proud of being in the *human family* and that the human family has to survive. When he included the human family in his remarks, he extended his advice from Indigenous individuals and communities to all people, suggesting that this healing process is transcultural and basic to *all* peoples. Healing goes beyond the surface, beyond even cultural differences, to the core of what it means to be human and to be a member of the human family.

Albert Lightning, a chief, Elder and medicine man from the Ermineskin Band in Hobbema, Alberta (now Maskwacis), spoke to a gathering in Whitehorse, Yukon, in 1980 in full chieftain regalia. His message was that Indigenous culture had survived over the years because of the people's knowledge of Spirit. He called for a renewing of this ancient wisdom, saying that a core group of facilitators should be trained to work in a transcultural way with Indigenous communities to remind them of their Inner Being.

A participant brought the following prose poem to a personal development workshop to read in the morning circle. The poem affirms the place and role of Spirit in the healing process.

> *Spirit is the part of us that responds to beauty and goodness, who inspires us to give of ourselves, who calls us together and draws us away for peaceful reflection. The Spirit is the place where hope flutters its transparent wings, the gentle place where the candle of life steadfastly burns, the green place that nurtures love, the dark place that harbours grief.*
>
> *Spirit is the quiet place where we can be alone with our belief in the Creator, and it is from this place of compassion that we can reach out to others. Our Spirits join us together, even when we are strangers, and give us the words to speak to each other. Our Spirits lift us above the ordinary and open our eyes to even the smallest wonders. Spirit is the painter, the dancer, the teacher, the healer, the lover, the dreamer that lies within each of us.*
>
> — Anonymous

When individuals rediscover and claim their Spirit, they become *in-powered*. All true feelings of self-esteem and self-love, as well as all lasting motivation for change, come from this internal source. This re-connection with the Inner Self/Spirit provides individuals with a storehouse of self-knowledge, inner wisdom and personal power. The seers, healers, dreamers and warriors of long ago are *still* present. Reconnection with their Spirit enables them to disconnect from negative self-images and behaviours and, thereby, reconnect with others in positive, healing ways.

Because of the interactive nature of the individual and of the community, when individuals begin to heal, so do the invisible webs of community. Changes in one individual set in motion a new dynamic with all the other individuals to whom that person is connected. The interactional pattern is changed, and new, healing responses emerge.

It is also true that when individuals learn to love themselves by going through a healing process, they know the path that others will need to walk in order to heal. This is not to say that they are all-wise or that they can do the healing for another person, but they are now more aware of others because they are more aware of themselves.

It is generally true that the *process* of healing is similar for all individuals. It is in this way that individuals in the process of healing can become helpers for others. It is a heightened awareness of one's own self that enables the ability to *be* with another person in a helpful manner. To assume responsibility for one's own healing and growth, to analyze the process and to generalize from one's self to others is a powerful healing force in a community.

This is experiential learning at its most basic. An individual's ability to say, "I know who I am and I love me" is the bottom line of community healing. It radiates out from there to partners, family and community members.

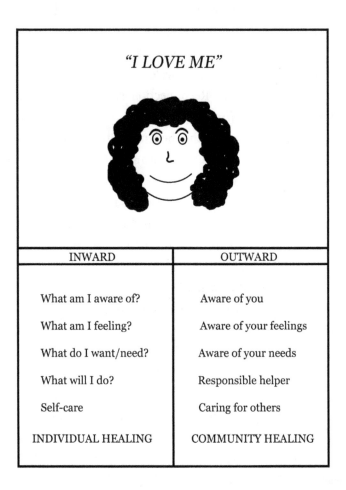

"I LOVE ME"

INWARD	OUTWARD
What am I aware of?	Aware of you
What am I feeling?	Aware of your feelings
What do I want/need?	Aware of your needs
What will I do?	Responsible helper
Self-care	Caring for others
INDIVIDUAL HEALING	COMMUNITY HEALING

Figure 7 "Self-Love Turned Inward, Outward = Healing Behaviours"

This overview of how individuals and communities become unwell and then can become well again forms the rationale for this model of transcultural community healing.

CHAPTER 3

BAJIC BELIEFJ OF THE TRANJCULTURAL MODEL

"Healing is a shared human journey."

THE TRANSCULTURAL HEALING Model emerged slowly over time as I worked with individuals, groups, organizations and communities. At the request of community people themselves, the focus of workshops transitioned from the community development ones to workshops more directly focused on personal issues.

When a group or organization requested a workshop of some type, it was always tailored to fit the stated needs and goals of the sponsoring organization or group, using the community development way of working.

Over time, workshops were added on topics such as death and dying, dealing with stress, communications, parenting, group dynamics, leadership, staff development, and alcohol and drug abuse. I began to start each workshop, no matter the focus, with a segment on self-awareness, asking them to answer the question, "Who am I?" The sharing of their answers always changed the group atmosphere from guardedness to togetherness and also reinforced the idea that all healing starts with *me*.

HEALING AS A SHARED HUMAN JOURNEY

As a non-Aboriginal, I felt that it was important for me not to tread on traditional cultural and spiritual beliefs. I learned that I must come to these encounters not as a teacher nor as an authority, nor as what used to be called "a wannabe Indian," but as myself, a human being on a personal journey.

I learned this for myself in a very dramatic way. While I was conducting a workshop in a northern community under contract to Grant McEwan College, the local medicine woman stopped by the workshop to check me out. When I passed her inspection, she informed me that if I was going to be working in Indigenous communities, I needed to be given a naming ceremony. She told me what coloured cloth to purchase for the ceremony. I was instructed to bring food that I had prepared myself. I felt privileged to be given this honour and did everything as she instructed. I even caught a fish, cooked it and brought all the required items to her camp on the appointed day. I was given a lunch of deer stew and then waited while she made the final preparations for the ceremony.

However, while waiting, I realized with a shock that my monthly period had started. I knew that this meant that I could not attend the ceremony. When I informed the medicine woman of my dilemma, she invited me to her teepee. She needed someone to listen to her because she had heavy burdens to carry, and we had a little healing ceremony, white-style. She rescheduled the ceremony for a later date. The same thing happened three times.

I began to realize that I was in the midst of learning a very important lesson, one that even the medicine woman had not intended to teach me. My Inner Self/Spirit was teaching me that I needed to remain within my own culture, while respecting and honouring her culture. Together, healing ways could be forged. I had wisdom to share about my journey; she had wisdom to share about her journey. This happening was an experiential learning for me in a transcultural microcosm.

That learning was an important one in my ongoing search for how to work effectively across cultures. It became a search about what it means to be a human being, how humans grow and develop and what kind of therapeutic environment is needed so that healing and growth can best take place.

Most psychologists would say then that to be whole or healed is to be in a state of balance between various aspects of one's body and mind. To be out of balance, in any one aspect, causes stress and, if not corrected, can become the genesis of disease. Therefore, to them, healing involves dealing with the causal factors that lie below the presenting symptoms, a process in which an individual returns to a condition that could be called normal. The range of their study of human behaviour goes from the abnormal to the normal—an illness model.

CHANGING THE FOCUS FROM ILLNESS TO WELLNESS

Some transpersonal psychologists like Carl Rogers, Abraham Maslow and Carl Jung have insisted that this return-to-normal emphasis is in error, that *normal* is to define what it means to be human from the perspective of a *disease model*—what is not normal. They have argued that true healing is a process that goes beyond normal functioning to a *wellness model*. They wanted to work with human beings at their highest potential, rather than at their lowest.

They came to believe that within each person is a seed, a blueprint of the person they can become. Becoming this person is an unfolding over time of becoming a unique human being.

Jung wrote extensively about the process of becoming a separate, indivisible whole. He said he knew about this process because his entire life was one of his own self-realization.

This process has been called various names: *Self-Actualization, Becoming All That One Is, Individuation, Self-Realization, and a Fully Functioning Person.* The healing as outlined by these giants in transpersonal psychology is, I believe, synonymous with the Indigenous Elders' belief that individuals need to rediscover and reclaim their *Spirit.*

It is very interesting that Carl Jung spent time in a Navajo tribe learning about their spiritual and cultural beliefs. In fact, they gave him the name Bear. Abraham Maslow also learned from Indigenous people; he spent several summers researching his theory of dominance in the Northern Blackfoot Indian Reserve in Alberta.

TO BE WHOLE IS TO BE IN A STATE OF BALANCE

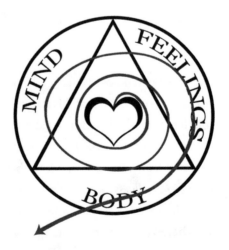

Figure 8 "Wholeness is Being in a State of Balance: Body, Mind, Feelings & Spirit"

Therefore, the commonality that runs throughout all these theories of healing, whether one is listening to Indigenous Elders, transpersonal psychologists or many of the world's philosophers and spiritual leaders, is the truth that each person has an Inner Self, a Spirit, and that to be whole is to be in a state of balance with one's inner and outer being.

Figure 8 depicts a state of being, a balance between all aspects of oneself—body, mind, and feelings. The heart in the middle of the circle represents, of course, the Inner Self/Spirit, that intangible being that lies at the core of the individual and at the core of the healing process. This Inner Self/Spirit is always deep within but becomes buried by life's negative happenings. The spiral represents the energy that is released from the Inner Self/Spirit for the healing process and illustrates the dynamic and inherent nature of healing.

THE STATE OF BALANCE BECOMES UNBALANCED

Everything that happens to an individual from the time he or she is conceived has an impact on this balance, either positively or negatively. Negative impacts create corresponding negative feelings such as anger, hatred or fear, depending on the situation. However, these feelings are usually not socially or culturally acceptable and are buried deep in the unconscious. The more destructive the environment a person is born into, the more negativity gets stored up within one's being. A child develops coping behaviours to deal with these negative feelings.

Often, coping behaviours that worked for a child become dysfunctional to oneself and others in adulthood. As one of my Gestalt teachers used to say, "Every emotion has a corresponding motion." Negative feelings produce negative behaviours. In addition, dysfunctional behaviours only serve to reinforce the negative feelings. The individual becomes trapped within these circular, self-fulfilling behaviours and feelings and, while Spirit still lies within, the individual becomes deeply alienated from it, from their Inner Self/Spirit. This alienation is depicted in Figure 9.

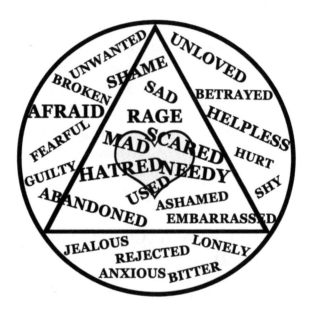

Figure 9 "Negative Feelings Block Individuals from Knowing Inner Self/Spirit"

Therefore, community healing begins with individual healing. Healing for an individual involves two basic stages: awakening to and claiming the Inner Self/Spirit, and dealing with negative feelings and behaviours from the past that prevent the individual from being who he or she really is. When healing is done in a group, the effects are multiplied as new healing ways of being with self and others emerge. A renewed community has begun.

THE MODEL: A SYNTHESIS OF COMMUNITY DEVELOPMENT, TRANSPERSONAL PSYCHOLOGY AND INDIGENOUS SPIRITUAL PRINCIPLES

The following points attempt to bring together the principles of community development, the work of transpersonal psychologists and the underlying spiritual principles of Indigenous culture. These comprise the basic beliefs and practices of the Transcultural Community Healing model.

▶ *Within all humans is a desire for personal transformation, the journey to becoming all of what one "is."*

▶ *Being whole involves a balance in mind, body, feelings and Spirit.*

▶ *An Inner Self/Spirit is the source of internal wisdom and is the motivating force for healing and growth.*

▶ *This Spirit is still present, despite whatever destructive things have happened to an individual.*

▶ *Negative things that have happened to individuals determine how they feel about themselves and are the source of negative behaviours towards oneself and others.*

▶ *Negative feelings and memories, especially those from early childhood, are usually buried deeply in the unconscious; these must be revisited, brought to consciousness and dealt with.*

▶ *Healing is a calling forth and remembering of the Inner Self/Spirit and aligning the everyday self with the higher Self.*

▶ *Individuals need a safe, caring, non-judgmental group envi-ronment in which to heal, to discover their Inner Self and to work with the issues that keep them from being who they are.*

▶ *Individual healing in an experiential workshop vastly mul-tiplies the possibilities for personal healing and results in healing relationships between participants.*

▶ *A strong support group is formed whose members have the tools for, and are committed to, ongoing healing.*

▶ *There is a direct relationship between the healing of indi-viduals and community healing. When individuals return to their everyday lives, all their relationships are presented with a role model, a catalyst for the transformation of others.*

▶ *Introducing this kind of healing into the larger community causes disruption of relationships, because individuals have changed behaviour. Great pressure is often put on individ-uals to return to their former way of being. If individuals remain true to their new learnings, steadfastness itself is a powerful dynamic for change.*

▶ *As individuals, their relationships and their small groups begin to heal, the larger community will begin to reflect those new healing ways of "being and doing." It is a grassroots, transpersonal, transcultural transformational process.*

While the Transcultural Community Healing Model deals with psychological and spiritual issues, there is no teaching of any specific religious, cultural or spiritual beliefs. As part of their healing, participants in the Healing Circles are encouraged to explore their own attitudes, beliefs and behaviours in relation to their spiritual practices.

CHAPTER 4

HEALING CIRCLES

"All real learning is Self-discovery."

THIS MODEL PROPOSES a series of experiential workshops for community healing—personal, inter-personal, small group, and community. While each Healing Circle in the model focuses on a different aspect of overall community healing, all circles use an experiential learning format.

EXPERIENTIAL LEARNING

Experiential learning is experience-based self-discovery. In this case, the self-discovery takes place within a group setting. An experiential workshop is designed specifically to be a living laboratory where the subject of study is primarily one's Self. An experiential workshop is not an artificial situation; it is a simplified and concentrated slice of life.

Ways of being, inside and outside a workshop, are basically the same. Behaviours reflect how individuals feel about themselves, and how they feel about themselves in relationship to others and to their environment. To become aware of these patterns is the first step in healing. Without awareness, no healing is possible, nor can a person make a choice to change behaviours.

People carry within themselves all their learned ways of being and doing, and they react to any new situation with the same feelings and coping mechanisms that they have learned since birth. Nothing is meaningless; everything an individual feels, does, says, thinks, dreams of, or knows is a statement about themselves. Some of these ways of being and doing are healthy; some are unhealthy; almost all are automatic, unconscious reactions. Most people go through life on automatic pilot, mindlessly reacting to events, never aware of *why* they feel or act in a certain way.

In an experiential workshop, the individuals use themselves as their own textbook, the group as their learning environment, and the workshop facilitator as a guide, but not an authority. Personal healing is not something that is done to a person from the outside in, but a process that starts from the inside out. It is not an easy process.

FACILITATING EXPERIENTIAL WORKSHOPS

When I was first beginning my work in Aboriginal communities, I was struggling with how to facilitate an educational experience in a nontraditional teaching way. One night, I had an important dream that taught me how to be a facilitator of Healing Circles and how to work with others at a transpersonal and spiritual level. The Teaching Dream went as follows.

I was trying to explain my community work to someone. The person I was talking to said that I should turn on a tape recorder while I was explaining my work. He said that not only would my words and thinking be clarified as I heard myself talking, but that the tape could be used to enable other helpers know the direction they could take when working in communities.

As I began to talk into this tape recorder, I saw that I was in a room with a group of people, but the people were old-fashioned wardrobes. In each wardrobe, much information, knowledge and wisdom had been stored. Yet, the wardrobes were lying on their backs and sides all over the room in many different directions, as if a hurricane had just gone through. Precious treasures, as well as garbage, food, papers, hangers, clothes—everything—were strewn in all directions.

I knew that it was now time for me to "do something," and I set about the task of cleaning up and "organizing" these wardrobes! I thought that it was up to me to provide the information and the skills and perhaps the motivation necessary to restore order to the scene.

*A voice corrected me, saying, "Stop! Look again!" As I looked more closely, I realized that I was **not** cleaning up or organizing or motivating or teaching. In fact, it looked like I was "doing nothing." I was standing in the middle of the room. In my hands were multitudes of shining, transparent webs, each one coming from the inside of a wardrobe. As I activated the strings and pulled on them, they glistened in the bright light and became more visible. The more I pulled out the shining strands, the more the wardrobes began to sort themselves.*

As if by magic, clothes went on hangers and were hung in the wardrobe; garbage went in trash containers; papers returned to their proper folders; folders lined up in sequence. There was a flurry of activity happening "all by itself." When order had been restored, each wardrobe stood

up and, with the others, formed a circle. I walked from the
center to become just another member of the circle.

This dream captured not only the philosophy and theory behind the Transcultural model but the method that can be used
to work in a community if one actually respects the idea that
everything needed by individuals and communities to heal lies
within themselves, not in the facilitator.

In experiential workshops, exercises are specifically designed
to engage an individual's whole Self within a group setting *on
a specific issue*, inviting them to become aware of what is happening. The invisible strands of awareness that are activated
makes what has been invisible become visible. When a person
sees what has been invisible, becoming conscious of something
that they have been unaware of previously, the totality of their
whole being is involved: body, feelings, mind and spirit. It is
not just a thinking event; it is a wholistic happening. I believe
that this educational method is compatible with the traditional
Indigenous way of learning by doing. It is vastly different from
the traditional lecture format within which a teacher/authority
presents information to students.

OVERALL STRUCTURE OF AN EXPERIENTIAL WORKSHOP

The format is not set in stone, to be followed rigidly. An experiential workshop flows like a river. No two facilitators will
guide the river raft in exactly the same manner, nor will the
group's issues always be the same. Yet, the facilitator should *know*
the overall purpose of each Healing Circle and the exercises introduced to reach that purpose. This *knowing* is the compass that

gently keeps the group's process flowing in the general direction, being alert to unintended opportunities for healing moments.

No matter how many years of experience the facilitator has, it's important to prepare carefully for every workshop. Keeping in mind the goals and the reasoning behind each of the exercises, their sequencing and their structure should be reviewed. In this way, one can adapt to what is needed in the moment—to add, subtract or alter the agenda.

An experiential workshop has a rhythm. It should start out slowly, ensuring that everyone understands the goals and feels comfortable enough to be open to whatever comes next. The middle part of the workshop gains momentum as the exercises are processed, awarenesses are heightened and feelings are expressed. The closing should bring the emotional level back down by helping people think about what has just been experienced. So, in brief, the rhythm goes: head, heart, head. Or head, feelings, head.

The preparation of the *space* for a Healing Circle is a time in which the facilitator's role also includes inner space preparation, in order to be ready for the role of facilitator. Getting ready is a meditative experience, becoming quiet and in tune with oneself. It is also a time to get *connected* with a co-facilitator, if there is one. It is vital for co-facilitators to be in harmony and peace with each other because group members can sense and react to tension between co-leaders. Ensuring that there is plenty of lead time for room preparation and *centering* is important because, in essence, as soon as the first participants arrive, the workshop has begun.

It is important that the room looks welcoming, colourful and comfortable. As soon as people come through the door, they should sense that *something* is different. Room arrangement includes:

- ▶ Flip chart sheet with the specific name of the Healing Circle, the drawing that represents that specific circle, the dates of the workshop and name of the facilitator

- ▶ Flip chart sheet listing the goals of the Healing Circle

- ▶ Circle of chairs, with journals, box of felt-tip pens, pens or pencils

- ▶ Candle on a tray in middle of the circle, matches

- ▶ Table for sign-in sheet, nametags, supplies, display books

- ▶ List of supplies needed for specific Healing Circles

- ▶ CD player and CDs—music should be playing softly when people arrive

It is crucial to ensure a safe, caring environment for participants. It is when people feel *safe* that their defences come down and they become open to change. That way, the energy participants usually use in groups to present an acceptable mask to others is available to examine what is happening right here, right now.

Participants are encouraged to be real and to look at themselves honestly, no matter what they discover. This encouragement, of course, is within a safe environment of workshop guidelines, agreed upon by the group. There are no pre-set ways of responding, nor right answers, just increased awareness about what is happening in the moment to oneself and to others. Awarenesses and their accompanying feelings are shared with the group without judgment.

This non-judging aspect is crucial, as it allows individuals the opportunity to admit to themselves, and to others, what they are really feeling and doing. Non-judgment does not mean condoning; non-judgment gives individuals the *space* in which they can be real and authentic, sometimes for the first time.

Each day should have an opening and closing ceremony. In the morning, the lighting of the candle and an inspirational poem, prayer, or smudging brings participants' attention to being in the now. A suggestion for an inspirational poem with which to start the workshop is provided in each format. However, thereafter ask for a volunteer to select something to share. It is good to have a variety of books on the display table from which to choose. These daily choices are added to the after-workshop write-ups for the journals.

Each morning, with the exception of the opening session, a circle go-round called "Where am I?" asks participants to go inward and become aware of what they are feeling, experiencing or wondering about. They share this awareness in one sentence, starting with "I." These statements help bring participants to the *now*; however, what people say is not processed at this time. They give the facilitator a snapshot of where the group is and what needs to be tended to at some point.

As participants work individually and in groups on the experiential exercises, the opportunities for growth are multiplied many-fold. As one participant shares with the group, others who have had similar experiences are also making their own personal connections. Each person's sharing affects the whole group, and what is happening in the whole group, in turn, affects the individual. A synchronicity takes place as individuals become more comfortable and open with one another. It is then that many unplanned, spontaneous things happen.

It is not enough just to have an experience, important as that is. In the final stage of an experiential workshop, it is crucial that individuals and groups get closure concerning the segment of work that has just been completed. New awarenesses need to be reinforced at a rational, conscious level. To answer the question of what have they learned about themselves and what they will they do differently now broadens conscious awareness of their own process and enables the community webs to be strengthened.

The end of each day should be designed to bring closure to the day's activities. A closing ceremony is important—a circle, perhaps a one-word statement about the workshop experience or whatever seems to fit in order to disengage from the intensity of the workshop and from the group. One must turn one's attention from inner to outer realities, applying the new learnings and ways of being to the "back home" situation. This should be followed by the ritual of extinguishing the candle and some type of group connection: handshakes, hugs, whatever seems appropriate.

Evenings can be used in a variety of ways. At times, an extra workshop session may be required to finish the day's agenda. It is important to have downtime as well. Relaxed group time promotes feelings of belonging. Participants should be encouraged to spend some time alone, recording their experiences and their new awarenesses in their journal. Participants can be encouraged to bring musical instruments, have storytelling sessions, or be prepared to share some other talent or skill. Evenings are a good time to have sessions on self-care, perhaps learning about and practising massage. Eating together or planning a feast is always a good way to spend the last evening of the workshop.

After each day's work, it is important that the facilitator spend time alone, or with a co-facilitator, reviewing what happened in the group, who or what might need extra attention and how to proceed the next day. In this way, how much can be accomplished each day is tailored to the specific group and adjusted as the workshop evolves and specific needs arise.

Following the workshop, the facilitator should make up a packet to be sent to circle members, requesting that the packet be added to the workshop journals. The packet will include:

- ▶ Name and contact numbers of circle members

- ▶ All the flip chart information and inspirational material, e.g., poems

- ▶ Summary of the evaluations

In addition, the facilitator should submit to the planning committee a short summary of how the Healing Circle went, with observations and suggestions for improved planning. However, this report should not include any personal information on circle members. Confidentiality must be maintained at all levels.

THE CIRCLE OF HEALING: AN EXPERIENTIAL AWARENESS GUIDE

When individuals are involved in a healing process, *everything* that happens to them is potentially a healing moment, no matter the issue. The Circle of Healing is an awareness tool; if used effectively, it can provide a road map to move from an unconscious reaction to an event in one's life to making a conscious choice for healing and for changed behaviour. Each time around the Healing Circle is called a *gestalt*—finishing what was started. In the process, a person moves from the unknown to the known, the unconscious to the conscious. It facilitates an individual's understanding of where they are and what they need to deal with next when working on a specific issue.

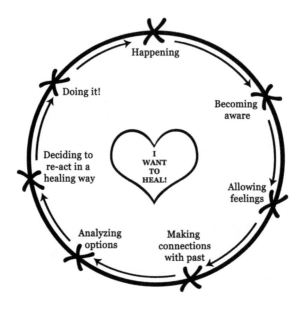

Figure 10 "Circle of Healing"

Real healing requires many trips around this circle, but if the Healing Circle is applied, not only in a workshop setting but also in everyday life, the process becomes second nature. Following the Healing Circle can become an exciting adventure, paying attention to each of the following stages:

I want to heal. In order to heal, a person must have at their core a deep desire and conscious *intention* to heal their life. *Intentionality* is not a last-minute New Year's resolution, quickly abandoned, but results from a deep, sometimes unconscious, unhappiness with some aspects or the totality of one's life. This produces a heartfelt desire for change. *Intentionality* produces an invisible force that underlies and often sets in motion personal growth and healing.

Becoming Aware of a Happening. Awareness is the first step along the path to healing. When, in life or in a workshop, something happens that triggers feelings and/or automatic, unthinking responses, people are often unaware of what is happening because they have buried these feelings and memories in the unconscious. These people are sleepwalking through life, subject therefore to automatic, habitual reactions to self and others. These automatic reactions are probably programmed in early childhood.

To change one's reactions and behaviours, one must first *become aware* that something *is* happening. Becoming aware is not an easy process, nor a comfortable one. It is like waking up from a deep sleep. Awareness opens the door to deeply buried feelings and memories that are often painful. To progress further on the healing pathway, one must welcome the awareness rather than slamming the door shut again.

Allowing Feelings to Emerge. Instead of repressing the emerging feelings, participants are encouraged to *allow the actual feelings to be expressed fully and uncensored.* Feelings are not rational; they are messy and are usually avoided, but at a cost to the healing process. People have developed many coping mechanisms to avoid feelings, especially the ones that originated in early painful childhood episodes. Deeply buried feelings must re-emerge and be released in a safe environment. To cry, to express anger, to feel sadness, shame or grief is crucial. Usually people don't know why they are feeling the way they do; they just do.

Making Connections with the Past. As feelings are expressed fully, individuals will begin to remember *when* they felt that way before, and to *make the connection* as to how what has just happened is similar to a previous event, usually a traumatic one. This connecting with the past is often accompanied with an "Aha! Now I get it" reaction. The light of understanding has penetrated the darkness of the unconscious, and the person will begin to understand why they are acting or behaving in a certain way.

Analyzing Options. Only after feelings are expressed and connections are made with the past does some degree of understanding take place. Now, thinking is not muddled with the repressed emotion, and a person can begin to *analyze* the situation. Various options on how to respond in a positive, growth-producing way can be considered.

Deciding to React in a Healthy Way. After weighing pros and cons of various options carefully, a conscious decision can be made to replace the former automatic, and unhealthy, reaction with a *healthy response*. This decision should be very specific. "The next time 'x' happens, this is what I *will* do; this is how I *will* react." To say "I will do" rather than "I wish to do" is powerful, because it engages one's willpower, the motivation to carry through on one's decision. Many people make good decisions for change at this point, but do not follow through. It is easier to think about changing one's behaviour than actually doing it.

Doing It. The real test, of course, is to complete the process by action; one must *do it*. In the doing, individuals become creators, or at least co-creators, of the events that make up their lives. They no longer are victims—of others nor of their past—because they have made a choice. They have become consciously "response-able." In this manner, step-by-step and event-by-event, they are regaining their personal power, the ability to say, "I am responsible for myself and my actions." Doing it can be practised in the safety of a workshop so that when participants return to their family and their community, they are better prepared to carry through on their decisions.

While seemingly simple, this Circle of Healing is a powerful tool. When a person is first learning how to use this awareness-to-action process, it will feel cumbersome and awkward. However, the more one works with it, the more it becomes almost automatic. Using it enables individuals to continue their healing process outside of the workshop setting. They become their own healers. Everything that happens then becomes an opportunity for learning, healing, self-responsibility and personal growth. This is a powerful life stance, because once individuals become fully responsible for themselves, they know how to be with others in healing ways.

FACILITATORS OF EXPERIENTIAL WORKSHOPS

The role of a facilitator is truly one of *facilitating*, as opposed to being a teacher or a decision-maker. In a helping relationship, all people have the need to be seen, heard and respected. It requires that the facilitator, Indigenous or non-Indigenous, be comfortable with different cultural realities, while respecting one's own. The individual being helped needs to know that their deepest fears and vulnerabilities can be revealed and explored and that their hurt and pain can be expressed and processed safely without judgment. It is a relationship where a person can come to terms with their own value system. In so doing, one's highest Self/Spirit is addressed, and this gives meaning, purpose and direction to one's existence. It is a sacred relationship at a very deep level, where love and respect are given and received.

Persons selected for this facilitating role must have special personal and spiritual characteristics that make them role models for individual and community healing. There are certain fundamental abilities and skills required to do this sacred healing work.

▶ Facilitators must be doing their own personal inner work; they need to be in an ongoing process of healing. Facilitators can only help another person as far as they personally have gone in their own healing. One is able to see beyond the surface of other people because one has experienced one's own journey.

▶ Facilitators should see their work as being a sacred trust and act accordingly. They need to take care of their own personal needs *outside* the workshop setting. They never should *need* anything from a workshop participant, nor use them for personal gratification in any way whatsoever. This also includes *not needing approval and/or pats on the back* from participants. An experienced and aware facilitator knows whether they have done a good job.

▶ Facilitators need to exercise a lot of love, patience, intuition and faith in the process. It is only after venting feelings that real knowings emerge. A helper's role is to facilitate an individual's awareness concerning who they really are and what they are really feeling. The process enables participants to bring unconscious issues to consciousness.

▶ Facilitators need to trust an individual's own process, knowing that within each person lies truth that will emerge when needed. Facilitators should not take a participant further than they are able to go on their own;

otherwise, they might not be able to handle the depth of their feelings.

▶ Facilitators are mirrors for a client, reflecting back what they see, hear, and sense to facilitate an individual connecting with unconscious material. Challenges, however, should be made gently, i.e., "I wonder if…" Pronouncements about where a person is or what they are feeling are not helpful because even an experienced facilitator cannot possibly know for sure about another person's path. Moreover, even if they could, they would be short-circuiting a unit of self-healing. Non-judgmental listening is one of the most powerful gifts a facilitator can give a workshop participant.

▶ Facilitators, whether knowingly or not, become channels for energy. This energy is magnified in a group setting. Therefore, a facilitator needs to be centered and in balance when working with a group. It is the calmness and centeredness of the facilitator that enables participants to let go, knowing that they will be safe. Since a workshop really begins as soon as participants enter the room, facilitators and their workshop environment must be ready ahead of time with no last-minute or rushed arrangements.

▶ Facilitators should not try to take on the mantle of someone else or become part of another culture in order to relate; healing takes place when contact is made at the human level, person to person. Facilitators can share aspects of their own journey, when appropriate, to illustrate a point and/or to make contact. After all, we are all on the journey.

IN SUMMARY

Experiential workshops for healing are mini-laboratories where participants use themselves and the group for self-discovery, growth and healing. Participants begin to understand who they are, how they got that way, and how to change. The Circle of Healing is a powerful tool in this self-discovery and self-recovery process, in which people become aware of what is happening to themselves and others. In this process, they can change unconscious reactions to conscious choices about their way of being, their beliefs and their behaviours. When this self-discovery happens in a group, then the opportunities for personal and community healing are manifold.

Experiential workshops require a different kind of leader, one who works with awarenesses, trusting that what each person needs for healing lies within their own Self/Spirit. Kahlil Gibran wrote in his book *The Prophet*:

> *No man can reveal to you aught but that which already lies half asleep in the dawning of your knowledge [awareness]. The teacher gives not of his wisdom but rather of his faith and lovingness. If he is indeed wise, he does not bid you to enter the house of his wisdom but rather leads you to the threshold of your own mind.*

— Gibran, p. 56

CHAPTER 5

IMPLEMENTING THE MODEL

"Healing in groups creates Community."

THE TRANSCULTURAL MODEL

THE TRANSCULTURAL MODEL for Community Healing is composed of different levels of experiential workshops or Healing Circles. This model can be seen as a parachute, capable of delivering a variety of healing opportunities into a community that is in need of, and requesting, healing.

The parachute, depicted in Figure 11 on the following page, delivers four levels of Healing Circles:

▶ Personal Healing, Levels One and Two

▶ Interpersonal Healing

▶ Small Group Healing

▶ Community Healing

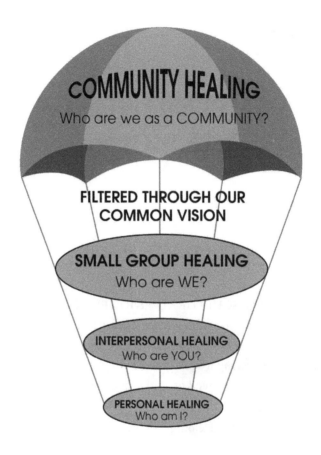

Figure 11 "Transcultural Model for Community Healing"

HEALING CIRCLES, FOUNDATION FOR COMMUNITY HEALING

The levels of Healing Circles outlined in the healing model attempt to address the brokenness of individuals within community, something often overlooked by community planners in the past. It seems self-evident to say that if a community is to heal, the individuals within that community must heal.

Individual healing is foundational to the healing of personal and community relationships. The broad underlying principles that are true for individual healing are also true at all levels of community and can be applied to other community programs. Over time, the healing principles could be incorporated into all community programming.

This model is not intended to replace the counselling programs that may already be in the community. However, since the model proposes that how people feel about themselves is at the root of all negative behaviours and addictions, the Personal and Interpersonal Healing Circles could be incorporated into specific treatment programs. This Transcultural model can be seen as the core of community healing.

When planning for all aspects of community healing is based on the principles and practices contained within the Transcultural Healing model, the micro level (the individual) and the macro (the community) work together toward the common goal of community healing.

When this healing is facilitated within a group setting, the Healing Circles become powerful change agents throughout the entire community and outward to the larger society. Individual healing begins (or continues) in the Personal Healing Circle; overall community healing begins as these individuals return to their everyday reality—their families, their significant relationships, their other small community groups and their workplace. Empowered with new discoveries about themselves and about the healing process, they will begin experimenting with new, or renewed, healthy behaviours.

Of course, applying these new learnings back home is, in itself, a learning and healing process. There will be successes and failures. As people who attend Alcoholics Anonymous meetings can testify, family and community members often resist an individual's changed behaviours, sometimes strongly. However, if failure can be viewed as part of the process and as a learning opportunity, then everything that happens from then on becomes an opportunity for healing. Support groups will emerge whose members are able to help others through difficult times. The healing potential becomes exponential, radiating out in all directions, magnified by the number of people in the circle and the number of significant relationships that each member has—and on and on and on.

WHAT ABOUT INDIGENOUS SPIRITUAL TEACHINGS AND PRACTICES?

What is being outlined here is a *process*, a way of working with individuals and groups. Being transcultural, it does not include a specific cultural component. There are several reasons for this. The most obvious one is that I, a non-Indigenous person, have developed the workshops that make up this model while working successfully for forty years in Indigenous communities and organizations.

I believe that the model provides a way of transcending cultural differences, while deeply respecting and honouring them. The process facilitates personal growth and healing within the cultural background of the participants. Using this model allows non-Indigenous persons to work in communities without falling into the trap of being one of those *outside others* whose goal is to missionize or to teach. It also allows Indigenous facilitators an alternative way of working with their own people and with non-Indigenous persons, truly a two-way street.

It has been my experience that when individuals begin to realize that they do have an Inner Self/Spirit, they usually are eager to continue their healing journey. As part of this journey, participants almost always have a great desire to learn more about, or to return to, their specific spiritual heritage. I have been told that individuals who want to learn about their cultural beliefs and practices must seek out and find their own Elder. The decision to search for a teacher of Indigenous knowledge and wisdom can be a powerful part of an individual's healing journey.

However, probably due to years of indoctrination in residential schools and the missionary efforts of various denominations on the reserves, some Indigenous people are hesitant, and even fearful, about participation in traditional cultural practices. There are differences among Indigenous people themselves regarding traditional ways and practices.

There are, however, common values and beliefs, which not only seem to span most Indigenous cultures in Canada, but also are compatible with the values and beliefs outlined in this healing model. These are:

- ▶ Belief in a Creator, a Higher Being

- ▶ The need to live in harmony with all of Creation—the whole

- ▶ Belief that everyone has a Spirit

- ▶ Inner ways of knowing

- ▶ The power of dreams and visions

- ▶ Values of wisdom, love, respect, bravery, honesty, humility and truth

► The power of the circle

► Consensus decision-making

► Learning by doing; teaching by example

In keeping with the philosophy of self-determination and the importance of personal choice in the healing process, an individual's decision about whether or not to return from the circle to specific Indigenous cultural practices and beliefs becomes a very crucial decision. Over the years of my career, I have seen many people choose to return; others have chosen to follow other spiritual paths or none at all. Whatever their choices are, the experiential workshops outlined in this model operate at a transcultural level, dealing with emotions, feelings and wisdom common to all who are members of the human family.

MULTI-LEVEL EXPERIENTIAL HEALING CIRCLES

The model works with multi-level Healing Circles, proceeding from individual healing to overall community healing. The healing principles learned in the first level apply to all the other levels, but with increasing complexity, moving from "Who am I?" to "Who are you?" to "Who are we?" and, finally, to "Who are we as a community?"

Individual and group exercises are specifically designed to reflect the focus of the different levels. As individuals become aware of, analyze and work through their feelings and issues at all of these levels, they cannot remain the same. They discover truths about themselves, about healthy relationships, about healthy group dynamics, and about what makes a healthy community. This is a transformational process.

PERSONAL HEALING CIRCLE, LEVELS ONE AND TWO

Since individual healing within a group setting is foundational to this Community Healing Model, both levels of the Personal Healing workshop should be implemented first, before any of the other levels. In fact, if a community could only provide one level of the model to its members, it should be the Personal Healing workshop. As mentioned before, this results in a core group of people who have bonded with each other and who are committed to personal and community healing. They will be the new change agents in the community.

In Levels One and Two, individuals will begin:

▶ To develop an awareness of each aspect of oneself (body, mind, feelings, spirit) and how these aspects relate to each other

▶ To recognize that each aspect has legitimate needs that must be recognized and taken care of if a person is to heal and to grow

▶ To realize that, no matter how hurt they are, they have an Inner Self/Spirit that has not been damaged

▶ To realize that the ability to say "I love me" is the basis for relating to self and others in a healing manner

▶ To deal with past traumas that created negative attitudes and behaviours

▶ To assume responsibility for themselves and their personal healing

▶ To realize that what is valid for one's personal growth is valid for others as well

▶ To create a strong support group with a sense of belonging

In the Personal Healing workshop, participants explore the fundamental question, "Who am I?" in a variety of ways. Personal Healing is divided into two parts: the first part focuses on the positive, the Inner Self/Spirit. The second part focuses on how negative events and traumas from the past prevent them from feeling positive about themselves.

In the first workshop, exercises are introduced in which they can identify their fears about being vulnerable, and guidelines are created to ensure that the circle will be a safe place. This need for safety is universal. All groups, Indigenous or non-Indigenous, have similar fears and develop similar guidelines. These form the foundation for the new ways of being in the subsequent workshops and, when practised, are healing for the community as well.

Participants are introduced to the concept that healing (to be whole) means to pay attention and to respect all aspects of one's Self: body, mind, feelings and Inner Self/Spirit. Following a visualization exercise, participants are asked to draw a picture, a symbol that represents this Inner Self. As participants begin to work with these images, some see for the first time that they are more than a bundle of negative emotions and behaviours. They often cannot believe, and even want to deny, that there is anything positive within, yet they have drawn something beautiful on paper which cannot be denied.

Slowly, they discover that they are more than they think they are, that they do have some part of themselves that is wise and that is in charge of orchestrating their healing. This process has the power to take individuals out of the thinking, hurting mode and into a more positive and intuitive aspect of themselves. As individuals work with and share these Spirit/Inner Self drawings, powerful connections take place between group members as they see themselves and others in a different light. They begin to see potential instead of problems.

In Level Two of the Personal Healing Circle, participants work on a traumatic event from their past, an emotional block that prevents them from being in tune with their Inner Self/Spirit. As individuals work on their issues, a variety of techniques and interventions are used to encourage the expression of deeply buried feelings; however, *the person is always in charge* of how much is shared. Talking about a past trauma is in itself a release, especially when others in the group are listening and empathizing. Many workshop participants have said, "No one has ever listened to me before. I have always been invisible." Participants are often amazed to realize that other people have gone through the same experience, and they no longer feel alone.

In both Level One and Two, comments from the other group members reinforce their new awarenesses and, again, cement bonds between members. Endings are always important. The circle is brought back to the positive—to remembering and re-inforcing Self/Spirit and sharing what behavioural changes they will make back home. Healing takes time; this circle is just the beginning of a long process.

However, participants now have new understandings and new ways of being. Returning home means doing it, the task of putting into practice every day their new, healthy way of being.

INTERPERSONAL HEALING CIRCLE

In the Interpersonal Healing workshop, individuals examine their way of being with others, positively or negatively, focusing on a significant person in their life. The workshop continues to reinforce the awareness that being whole requires the need to pay attention and care for all aspects of Self.

What has been learned about their own healing allows them to step back a bit, to see themselves in relation to others. Participants will be presented with a model that can be used to examine how they relate to a significant other and to understand how they can change the relationship in a healthy way.

The overall format will be similar to the Personal Healing Circle, regarding guidelines, housekeeping items, and the opening and closing ceremonies. Participants will begin:

► To reinforce their sense of who they are, as sacred beings with body, mind, feelings and spirit

► To explore their usual way of relating to others, especially in terms of significant relationships

► To learn how to change a relationship by changing personal attitudes and behaviours

► To practise healing ways of relating to others, including listening with an open heart

► To explore how the new awarenesses and behaviours can be applied to relationships at home and at work

► To continue to strengthen the bonds between group members, fostering feelings of belonging and community

SMALL GROUP HEALING CIRCLE

Whenever people come together in groups, certain things always begin to happen. Powerful, but invisible, webs are woven between participants who are often not aware of these dynamics. In the Small Group Healing Circle, these webs will be examined to answer the question: "What is happening among the group members?" and "How does what is happening affect the functioning of the group?" Again, the group is the textbook from which to learn about how groups function. This workshop can be adapted to any type of community group, whether the focus is on a family, staff development, or chief and council.

The overall format will be similar to the Personal Healing Circle re guidelines, housekeeping items, and the opening and closing ceremonies. Participants will begin:

▶ To reinforce their sense of who they are, sacred beings with body, mind, feelings and spirit

▶ To continue to build on and apply new awarenesses and behaviours from the first workshops

▶ To review how the group is organized to work together and what helps or hinders in terms of purpose, leadership styles, decision-making

▶ To learn more about each other's jobs and responsibilities

▶ To become a stronger group, fostering feelings of belonging and connectedness

▶ To apply what they have learned here about good working relationships to other groups in which they are involved

COMMUNITY HEALING CIRCLE

In the Community Healing Circle, community is defined as feeling connections between people—their shared values, desires and hopes. Community is people being self-responsible and yet responsible to others in interdependent relationships. It is sharing beliefs and ways of doing things that all (or most) agree on, including rules and regulations—the ways in which they are governed. Community is working together for the common good.

In the Community Healing workshop, the group will:

► Explore the meaning of community and the relationship between individual healing and community healing

► Create a vision for the future of the community

► Explore the question, "Who are we as a community— our shared values and beliefs?"

► Outline beginning steps to implement the vision, answering the question, "Where do we go from here?"

It is important to focus this workshop on the positive aspects of community, rather than the *what's wrong* approach. Working with a positive vision for the future not only provides the blueprint but generates the positive energy to move forward with planning for how to implement that vision. In this way, some of the negative aspects of community will be dealt with, as group members and community groups begin to discover more creative, positive ways to solve their community issues. In workshop jargon, this is a win-win situation.

Together, this series of workshops comprise a potent package for community healing that can be offered to a community that is in need of, and requesting, assistance. The vision developed for overall community healing can provide the framework for all subsequent decision-making. It can guide the restructuring of the community programming around common values, goals and methods for accomplishing those goals. The Community Vision provides the guidance for all community programing and decision-making, including social programs, educational and skill training, economic development and even infrastructure planning.

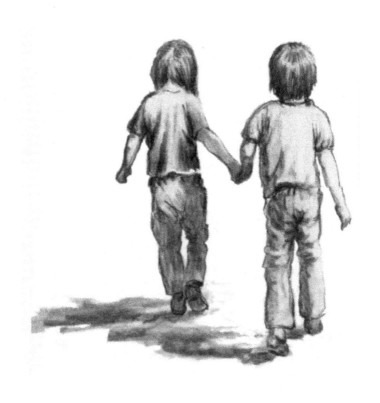

CHAPTER 6

JUGGEJTIONJ FOR PLANNING

"Planning→Implementation→Evaluation = Feedback Loop."

T HIS SERIES OF Healing Circles was designed to address a community's need for healing. The Healing Circles are based on transcultural principles that are a blend of community development philosophy, transpersonal psychology and Indigenous spiritual wisdom. Healing in the circle creates a new kind of community whose members are not only involved in their own healing, but are also gaining a common understanding of the healing process and creating support groups of like-minded people. The healing principles and ways of working, if adopted, can provide the foundation for and guide all community planning as well as the planning for these Healing Circles.

Peter Erasmus said that once you start with people involvement, community development [healing] is happening. Healing is not primarily a mental exercise. When people participate in an experience-based Healing Circle, their whole being becomes involved at many levels unless they choose to leave the group.

There is no one way to plan for such a serious undertaking as community healing. It is not the intention of this model, nor should it be, to outline a blueprint for implementation. Each community will need to undertake this task in its own way, remembering that there is no single right way. However, the importance of careful planning cannot be over-emphasized. The following section discusses some crucial aspects of planning which should be given careful consideration. These are not in any order of importance, but they are important!

COMMUNITY OWNERSHIP

The request for a healing process ideally should come from the community itself. The goal of any development or healing process is ownership of it by the people themselves; it must be their program. In any healing process, whether at the individual or at the community level, the first step is for people to become aware of and to acknowledge that something is wrong. An acknowledgement that something is wrong is the first step in healing and engages the desire and a willingness to do something about it. This means that some forward motion has already begun in individuals and the community. When the request for healing comes from the community, it has a chance of succeeding; too many programs imposed from outside have failed. An outside authority should not mandate healing programs; however, government can initially play a role by creating structures and resources that facilitate community healing.

TOP LEADERS AND DECISION-MAKERS ON BOARD

It is important that top-level community leaders and decision-makers be kept informed about and agree to the healing process if it is to evolve in all its healing power. If decision-makers do not understand and support the process, many roadblocks, intended and unintended, will occur.

Ideally, the chief and council should lead the way; they should be the first group to attend. In this way, they would not only set an example for the community members, but would emerge as a cohesive team with shared knowledge and experience about their own healing, as well as the community's.

There are additional benefits for the chief and council to be the first group. The task of the last circle, Community Healing, is to create a Community Vision and to answer the question, "Who are we as a people?" As they do this, underlying principles and values of the community are identified. It is out of this process that overall guidelines for future decision-making at *all* administrative levels can be formulated, thereby integrating traditional beliefs with a vision of the future.

Following the Community Healing workshop for chief and council, community members should be involved, adding their input to the above issues. The more people involved, the broader the impact and motivation for change.

PLANNING FOR IMPLEMENTATION OF HEALING CIRCLES

A planning team is needed to oversee the implementation of the model. An inter-departmental team would be ideal and would result in a wider sense of ownership of the process and responsibility for ensuring its success. The combined knowledge of an inter-departmental team concerning administrative affairs and community needs is important. The team's mandate should clearly outline the lines of authority, and then the team should be given as much autonomy as possible.

The delivery of these workshops to the staff can be structured in different ways, so as to bring staff members together in various combinations. Each way has its advantages and disadvantages. For instance, if all staff members from one department attend the series of Healing Circles together, this would result in an added benefit of staff development, team-building and organizational development, as well as personal healing. If staff members from different departments attend the series together, it will result in improved communication and cooperation between departments. Either way, there would be an added bonus of staff training and development.

That staff members could be expected to attend the circles as part of their job is not without precedent. In the 1970s, Native Counselling Services of Alberta developed a policy that every person who was hired had to attend an introductory workshop in personal awareness. Follow-up sessions were provided for those who wanted to continue their healing. The same kind of process was implemented for the Community Wellness Department of the Samson Band in Maskwacis, Alberta.

Another decision to make is about how and when to involve ordinary community members in the Healing Circles. Community members should not be mandated to attend. An individual must want to attend and make a choice to do so. Some people will not be ready, and this should be respected.

The scheduling of the Healing Circles and decisions about who attends, and when, should be thought through carefully. This can be done in several different ways:

▶ Chief and council alone

▶ Chief and council and department heads

► Staff members from one department

► Staff members from different departments

► Non-staff community members only

► Non-staff community members with staff members

Whatever the mix, attendance in a Healing Circle creates a mini-community, a support group whose members have an understanding of the healing process. In the end, a new foundation, a positive way of being, will have been experienced by all the adults in the community who choose to heal. It has been my experience that after attending a Healing Circle, individuals begin to work with their children and spouses, using some of the exercises and techniques from the workshops. In this way, each experiential workshop has multiple outcomes, the effects of each spreading out beyond the circle.

SUGGESTIONS FOR STRUCTURING HEALING CIRCLES

The best results are gained when:

► The expectations and goals for each session are clarified and agreed on by all stakeholders: chief and council, the planning team and the facilitator. Clear lines of communication and authority are needed. Who is in charge? Who makes the arrangements? The planning team should make all the arrangements in consultation with the facilitator. The facilitator should only need to show up, facilitate the workshop and provide feedback to the planning team.

▶ Individuals who are band employees should be free to be themselves when attending the Healing Circles without repercussions back on the job. Not only are the Healing Circles confidential, but a formal agreement should be made between the staff member and the planning committee that their job will not be affected by whatever they do or say in the Healing Circles.

▶ Ideally, the venue should be a hotel or lodge away from the community. A rural setting near water or the mountains brings an added dimension. Of course, wholesome food and congenial hosts are vital. The group room itself should feel welcoming. A fireplace and a rug always add to the ambiance as well as the comfort of the participants.

▶ Participants should know what to expect before they arrive. A brochure outlining workshop expectations should be provided, including the name of the workshop, the goals, the location, the dates, the travel arrangements, and any costs associated with it. In addition, a further explanation could go something like this: *A Healing Circle is a time for you to answer the questions: Who am I? How do I feel about myself? How can I heal my relationships, my groups and our community? Other individuals, like you, will join in the circle to search for answers to these questions. The facilitator's job is to help you to talk about yourself and your feelings and to ensure that the circle is a safe place to be. You will begin to see yourself—and others—in new ways, and you will find healthy ways of dealing with the issues in your life.*

▶ Each circle should be at least three days in length; five days is better, especially for the Personal Healing ones. The circles should be limited to eight to ten people to maximize the amount of time for each participant to do their work in the circle. Everyone in the room needs to be a participant—no watchers, observers, visitors or interruptions, except in an emergency.

▶ Participants are asked to keep a personal journal for each of the circles. These journals become personalized textbooks; they are invaluable in reinforcing the healing that takes place during the sessions. Participants usually treasure them, often rereading them when they are dealing with some crucial issue back home.

▶ Following the workshop, copies of all data generated in the workshop should be compiled and provided to the participants in booklet form, with a request that they add them to their journals. This includes copies of the inspirational readings, all flip chart material, a summarized copy of the evaluations, and a list of workshop participants with their contact numbers.

FLEXIBLE TIME FRAMES AND FUNDING

Flexible time frames and funding are crucial. The community healing work should be seen as a long-term process with time frames based on actual ongoing needs, not predetermined. Funding should be adequate and flexible, able to adapt to changing needs. When Peter Erasmus was discussing community work, he said:

The problem as seen from the outside is that the process is time-consuming. It does not bring quick results. You can't seem to justify it dollar-wise. It takes time because it is, in essence, people-development. This involves a basic attitude change and the acquiring of new skills, knowledge and behaviours. These changes are difficult to evaluate and assess on any performance appraisal. This [healing] work should be recognized as being a long-term process.

– Erasmus, 1991, p. 11

ONGOING EVALUATIONS

Ongoing evaluation is a crucial part of implementing the healing model. Evaluations should guide the process and inform the next steps. Evaluations should not be an elaborate process; simple works best. Honest feedback is important; therefore, evaluations should not be seen as punitive, but be based on what is positive and what could be better.

There are at least three levels of evaluation: evaluation of each Healing Circle by the participants, evaluation of the overall implementation process by the planning committee, and evaluation of the work of the planning committee itself.

1. **Evaluation of Healing Circles**. A simple questionnaire can provide an efficient, accurate summation of how the participants experienced the workshop and any changes they would like to see. It could look like this:

   Name & Date of Workshop: _____
   Facilitator: _____

   ‣ Given the objectives, how would you rate your experience in this workshop? (Poor, Fair, Good, Very Good, Excellent)

   ‣ What session was most helpful to you?

> What would you like to have been done differently?

> How did you personally benefit from this workshop?

> What words come to mind when you think of this workshop?

> What other comments or suggestions do you have?

These unsigned questionnaires can be summarized easily. Cumulative records should be kept of the responses by type of workshop and by date. These findings provide the data to streamline the process and to inform the planning committee about any changes that may be needed to the workshop formats or to the overall implementation process. The comments from workshop participants are usually very insightful and relevant; they are an excellent way of getting honest and helpful feedback.

The facilitator should also submit a brief written assessment and any suggestions needed. This assessment should not disclose names or issues that a specific person dealt with because participants need to know that what happens in the workshop will not be used in any way without their permission.

2. **Evaluation of the Implementation Process.** The planning committee should evaluate periodically how the overall healing process is evolving, making changes as necessary. The following evaluation form can provide a quick overview. It is based in the overall principles of community development.

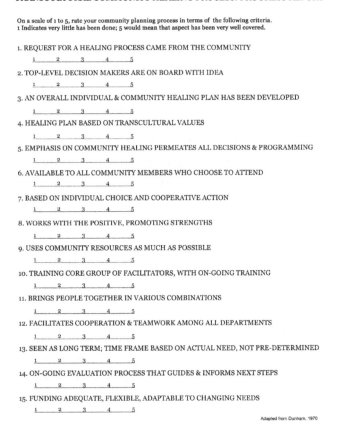

TRANSCULTURAL COMMUNITY HEALING PROCESS: PROGRESS REPORT

On a scale of 1 to 5, rate your community planning process in terms of the following criteria.
1 Indicates very little has been done; 5 would mean that aspect has been very well covered.

1. REQUEST FOR A HEALING PROCESS CAME FROM THE COMMUNITY
   1   2   3   4   5

2. TOP-LEVEL DECISION MAKERS ARE ON BOARD WITH IDEA
   1   2   3   4   5

3. AN OVERALL INDIVIDUAL & COMMUNITY HEALING PLAN HAS BEEN DEVELOPED
   1   2   3   4   5

4. HEALING PLAN BASED ON TRANSCULTURAL VALUES
   1   2   3   4   5

5. EMPHASIS ON COMMUNITY HEALING PERMEATES ALL DECISIONS & PROGRAMMING
   1   2   3   4   5

6. AVAILABLE TO ALL COMMUNITY MEMBERS WHO CHOOSE TO ATTEND
   1   2   3   4   5

7. BASED ON INDIVIDUAL CHOICE AND COOPERATIVE ACTION
   1   2   3   4   5

8. WORKS WITH THE POSITIVE, PROMOTING STRENGTHS
   1   2   3   4   5

9. USES COMMUNITY RESOURCES AS MUCH AS POSSIBLE
   1   2   3   4   5

10. TRAINING CORE GROUP OF FACILITATORS, WITH ON-GOING TRAINING
    1   2   3   4   5

11. BRINGS PEOPLE TOGETHER IN VARIOUS COMBINATIONS
    1   2   3   4   5

12. FACILITATES COOPERATION & TEAMWORK AMONG ALL DEPARTMENTS
    1   2   3   4   5

13. SEEN AS LONG TERM; TIME FRAME BASED ON ACTUAL NEED, NOT PRE-DETERMINED
    1   2   3   4   5

14. ON-GOING EVALUATION PROCESS THAT GUIDES & INFORMS NEXT STEPS
    1   2   3   4   5

15. FUNDING ADEQUATE, FLEXIBLE, ADAPTABLE TO CHANGING NEEDS
    1   2   3   4   5

Adapted from Dunham, 1970

3. **Evaluation of Progress and Process of Planning Committee's Sessions.** The planning community should evaluate their own process after each meeting. How did the meeting go? How satisfied were they that the goals for the session were accomplished? How did the members feel about the meeting? In this way, the planning committee itself becomes part of the healing process, as they learn ways to be open to new ideas, to listen to each other, to make collective decisions and to work for the good of the whole. Simple rituals at the beginning and

end of a session, like prayer or smudging, often set a positive tone for the meeting.

TRAINING A CORE GROUP OF FACILITATORS

Facilitators will be needed to conduct these Healing Circles. It has been my experience that there are many potential facilitators already in a community or in a neighboring community who would, with a little training, be capable of conducting these Healing Circles. Some may already be working in the human services field.

Careful selection of these potential facilitators is important. Look for mature community members who are already committed to their own healing journey. They should be persons who are seen as leaders and who are looked up to and respected. They walk their talk and have personal characteristics of integrity, respectfulness, honesty and openness. These ways of being are more important than academic qualifications.

However, a professional psychotherapist will be needed to train the facilitators. Professionals, whether psychologists, social workers, or nurses, are not all alike. They will not necessarily be in tune with this Transcultural model. Select a person to do this training of the facilitators who has all the personal qualities required when selecting the potential facilitators. In addition, the professional must be mature and have life experience, as well as have academic qualifications. Ideally, they have training in individual or group therapy. Such persons will have the ability to work in communities as equal partners, not as authority figures.

Training the facilitators should involve them having them participate as a group in all the Healing Circles: Personal,

Interpersonal, Group and Community. Participation in the circles should be supplemented with debriefing sessions to discuss group process, how things went, what could have been done differently, and what worked well. There should also be a segment on how and when to make appropriate referrals to other community resource agencies. The core group itself then becomes a community, using themselves and the group for their learning. As they do this, strong bonds are formed and a peer support group is created.

After this basic training, perhaps members of the core group could specialize in one type of workshop, thereby developing expertise in one specific area. Co-facilitating the Healing Circles, ongoing supervision, consultation and regular meetings with the core group would be important to the training. The members of the core group should be encouraged to attend other types of training, compatible with wholistic focus, to become as widely knowledgeable as possible.

Thinking on a larger scale, this core group could be multiplied many times over, and soon there would be a small army of trained helpers to go into communities, as needed.

CHAPTER 7

COMMUNITY VIJIONING: A CAJE JTUDY OF TAKU RIVER TLINGIT FIRJT NATION

With Louise Gordon, Spokesperson

"If you don't have a dream..."

T HE FOLLOWING CASE study is an example of what can happen when a community and its leaders are motivated to begin a healing process. It also discusses openly the failures that occurred and the reasons for these failures. It will be told in two parts: "Creating a Community Vision" and "The Rest of the Story." "The Rest of the Story" is written by Louise Gordon, Spokesperson for the Taku River Tlingit First Nation.

CREATING A COMMUNITY VISION

In 1985, my partner, Bob Langin, and I were invited to come to a small northern British Columbia band, at that time still called the Atlin Indian Band. The chief had just finished an alcohol treatment program and was very desirous of starting a healing program in his community. He, with the agreement of his band manager and council members, contracted with us for a community development workshop, with follow-up workshops to be determined.

This workshop was to be held for the chief and council and all staff members. They had outlined the goals of the workshop to be:

▶ To learn helpful ways to work in our community

▶ To learn helpful ways of communicating with each other

▶ To become a stronger team

▶ To learn about each other's jobs and responsibilities

▶ To learn how to help each other reach our goals

As most of the staff members were new to their jobs, they were not used to working together. It soon became obvious that they did not really know what their jobs were or what their goals should be. This made working together difficult; many misunderstandings and hard feelings were occurring on the job, and these were reflected in the community and in the workshop. Quite a bit of time was needed to create a comfortable and safe workshop environment, as well as to deal with their ongoing working relationships in the band office. However, the community development workshop quickly turned into a staff development, team-building exercise. The organizational chart was examined in concrete terms:

▶ Who reported to whom?

▶ Job descriptions, responsibilities and limitations

▶ Effective and ineffective lines of communication

▶ What staff members needed in order to do their jobs well

▶ How to work harmoniously together as a team

Interestingly, the band member who was at the lowest level of the official organizational chart, the janitor, was the community healer, medicine woman and wife of the chief. In actuality, the lowest was the highest.

In like manner, a seemingly simple group exercise that had been planned as an icebreaker and a way of bringing group members closer together turned out to be the most productive activity of this workshop. In the magical way that often happens in experiential workshops, a simple exercise turned into a potent planning activity; it became community development at its essence. Participants were asked to draw a picture, in colour, of how they would like to see their community ten years in the future.

One by one, as participants shared their drawings with the group, powerful word pictures emerged, identifying important cultural and community values and desires. They called this "The Invisible Community." They described happy people working and playing together, children learning from elders, the community as a watering hole summer and winter (meaning continual warm, positive feelings), fresh water washing the shores (hope for a new beginning), sunlight and rainbows, canoes tied together on the lake and passing tea and bannock back and forth, heavy equipment working, women tanning hides and a moose head roasting over a fire.

These images were symbolic of how they wanted to feel in their renewed community. The chief summed up their Invisible Community this way: "The feelings represented by these word pictures go back thirty to forty years ago. They go back to the way we were: a peaceful, loving people, working and playing and getting along with each other and with our neighbouring villages."

A discussion followed about how this Invisible Community could be translated into a Visible Community. They saw specific buildings and structures: a new Cultural Centre in the middle of the community, round, made of logs, with a blue roof. It would have a room for the Elders in the middle, with band offices around the center and a totem pole on the outside. There would be a year-round lodge, a learning centre with a craft room, a park across the lake, a marina, a snowshoe factory, a retreat centre for alcohol and drug rehabilitation, a community garden growing vegetables and flowers, and upgraded and spruced-up houses.

The activities they saw happening in their Visible Community were Elders at the Cultural Centre teaching the old ways, telling stories, serving tea, teaching native language, cultural cooking, tanning, sewing and beading. The chief, council, and band staff were working together for the future of the community and reaching out to make connections with the nearby communities.

In the Community Learning Centre, people were upgrading their education and learning new skills, i.e., heavy equipment training, carpentry, gardening. At the year-round Lodge, people were attending training workshops and conferences. Tourists were being taught about the local culture and being guided on hunting and fishing expeditions. Snowshoes were being produced and sold in the new factory.

The community development workshop had turned into staff development out of necessity; individuals did not know how to do their jobs nor how to work harmoniously with each other. This change of agenda was needed before the workshop could proceed with any planned community development activities.

Yet, the focus returned to community development due to the unplanned visioning exercise, illustrating the principle that individual and group work has to start where people actually are, not where the group leader wants them to be.

The chief and council, and staff, began to realize that they had a long, exciting road ahead, although none of the participants, including ourselves, realized how long the road was to be. They discussed how they would go about planning for these changes on a long-term basis and decided that they needed to develop guidelines for decision-making when turning their Vision into a concrete reality. Some of these guidelines were:

▶ The Creator guides our Elders; Elders guide our leaders.

▶ All community members are equal.

▶ The wellbeing of all community members must be the core of all community planning. This means people-centered decision-making, with community members involved at all levels.

▶ Planning must be action-oriented, getting things done the goal.

▶ Economic stability is a long-term goal—community self-sufficiency without government grants.

▶ People should be able to work at what they want to do and are good at, teaching each other.

▶ Community should return to cultural ways with a balance of old and new.

▶ There should be cooperation at all levels—community people, chief, council and all departments, inter-community, intra-community.

▶ It is crucial to help community members to know who they are and help them to be what they are.

▶ The Community Cultural Centre building and its activities should reflect our cultural beliefs.

In summing up the process, some of the group members had suggestions regarding improvements to the day-to-day procedures for conducting band business, especially the sharing of information regarding decision-making and more clarification regarding job expectations. Much of the summing up consisted of sharing insights regarding being on the team, such as:

▶ If you want something [our team] to be strong, you have to put something in.

▶ When we make a decision together, it makes us stronger as a team.

▶ A problem at home causes friction at work.

▶ When I am feeling down, I tell people so they are extra careful with me. We all feel better that way.

▶ My relationship with my wife is number one; my job is number two. If number one is out of order, it affects number two!

▶ Mistakes are one thing I am not afraid of now, because I will know there is no such thing as a person who does not make a mistake. We can learn from our mistakes.

► When you get something for nothing, you do not take care of it.

In this visionary process, new hope was kindled, misunderstandings and disagreements were resolved, and the chief and council, together with their staff, now had direction and a purpose. Following the workshop, they held a community campout for all community members. There, they planned to introduce the new Community Vision and engage them in the process of community building.

Following the campout, my partner and I moved to Alberta due to health concerns, and we had no further contact with the band. In 2016, when this book was being written, a series of synchronicities happened that brought Louise Gordon and myself together again. Many changes had taken place in the thirty-plus intervening years. The Atlin Indian Band was now the Taku River Tlingit First Nation, and Louise Gordon, band manager, was now the chief, or Spokesperson, as she would prefer to be called. She has graciously agreed to relate what changes have occurred in those intervening years, as well as what worked and what did not.

THE REST OF THE STORY

By Louise Gordon, Spokesperson—Taku River Tlingit First Nation

Way back in 1985, we sat down one night, looked at our community and realized that it was broken. I say "we" because Jenny Jack was actively working with our band at that time. She was head of the Land Claims Department and I was the band manager for administration. She was the manager for Lands. We just called it Lands at that time.

OUR COMMUNITY BEFORE THE COMMUNITY DEVELOPMENT WORKSHOP

We were trying to organize an administrative structure that would work for us. People, including us, were in a state of confusion. There was a lack of capacity, skills and know-how, and lack of funding to move forward. We had just started applying for funding for five new community workers: a Native National Alcohol and Drug Abuse Program (NNADAP) worker, an Indian Affairs worker (it was called Indian Affairs at that time), a social assistance worker, a community health worker and a community education liaison worker.

At a healing level, there were quite a few people still actively drinking in the community. At that time, there weren't many drugs; people hadn't been introduced to drugs, so they were drinking a lot. This resulted in violence and abuse—what we now are calling "lateral violence." Lateral violence means abuse that is passed from one person to another. Our chief had just sobered up and wanted to help others. (Our administrative leader was still called *chief* at that time, but that changed as a result of the process we started then.) We didn't know what to do, but we knew that we needed to heal. We needed to heal as a community together.

So we said, "We'll have a community development workshop." And that's what we did. What we did was to write a proposal, and we took it to this lady at Indian Affairs. I will always remember that day when we put in the proposal. She asked us, "How did you think of this?" We told her that we were just sitting down, wondering how we could move forward, and we realized that our community was broken.

We got ahold of some people from Whitehorse, Bob and Geneva. They had a company called Explorations Counselling & Training Services. They agreed that they would come down and conduct this workshop for us.

So they came down. We were just ready to start the workshop when the lady from Indian Affairs phoned me. She said, "What are you doing?" At that time, I didn't know that I was supposed to wait for us to sign the contribution agreement before going ahead with the workshop. So I said, "We are just about ready to start our community development workshop." And she said, "Oh my God! You were supposed to sign the contribution agreement first." I said, "You never told me that. You were supposed to be here last week, but you didn't show up. We have to move forward, and we are doing that. This is what we need." She said, "Well, I'll be right down!"

And two hours later, she was there with the contribution agreement in hand, and that was the beginning of our workshop. The contribution agreement was signed. So, it was clear that we weren't the only ones who were confused. Indian Affairs and our service providers were confused, too, and their confusion was passed down to us. That was the day I realized that much of the band's administrative confusion was really passed down to us by our funders. That's where it started. Later on, we worked on *that* piece, but that's how we started our community development workshop.

VISIONING OUR FUTURE: THE COMMUNITY DEVELOPMENT WORKSHOP

In the community development workshop, the visioning exercise we did was helpful; it was the seed that started things moving. The seed for community change was planted in 1985.

We drew pictures of what we would like our community to be in the future. We sat around and talked about what people really wanted in the community.

People talked about many things that they wanted, especially the warm feelings of community and togetherness that they remembered from long ago. They wanted to return to cultural ways and traditions and balance them with the new ways of doing things. Physically, people really wanted to build a Taku River First Nation government building because we were all working in little houses all over the place. We were growing so quickly that we had to expand our infrastructure. We had one little house for the land claims office. We had a bigger house for the social programs office. We had a band office that was already there. Administration, Capital Projects and the secretary were working out of the band office. We had tried to organize things so we could increase the services to our people, but we ran out of space.

The other priorities that people really wanted were a community garden and a hydro plant. Over the years, I had heard so many times that people wanted a garden. It became clear that a garden was a top priority.

I don't recall all that was talked about in the workshop, but working on health and healing for people was very important; building the administration building was important. Everybody having work was important. We talked about lots of things. Later, when I looked at past documents, leadership had often brought up the need for many of the same things.

VISIONING OUR FUTURE: LAND CLAIMS WORKSHOP

We had already filled out proposals for the health-related positions, the NNADAP, Community Health Representatives

(CHR) and social assistance. We got funding for two NNADAP workers and a CHR. The social assistance program at that time was actually administered by Indian Affairs. We later took over the administration of that program. We sent these people out for training before they went into those positions.

We filled out applications for other funding. The Lands manager, the chief and I, with help from a few other people, made the funding applications. We also filled out another comprehensive claims proposal to the federal government and, from the funds we were granted, we built on the community development workshop.

The whole community was invited to a campout in order to help us plan for the future of the Taku River Tlingits. We called this workshop "Land Claims." That was an idea from the Lands manager. Involving the whole community in the planning was once the foundation of our community. We were doing it that way again. It was held at the Five Mile Point Culture Camp.

The Elders who were sitting in that meeting looked at the title and said, "Land claims!" I still remember that moment. "We've got no land to claim. This is our land. We're not claiming any land. When you claim something, it's not yours to begin with. That's not what we're doing! What we need to do is to plan on how we're going to use this land and what parts of our land that we want to share."

So that's how our community-planning workshop started. It was unreal. The advice of the Elders was so important. When I heard the Elders speak, I knew then that we were going to start moving forward.

Most of the community came down to that workshop. We had a young man who worked like a beaver even though he had a disability. It was Down Syndrome. He wanted to help. We tied a moose head on a tripod over the fire and went away. When we came back, he was turning it like it was supposed to be turned. He became a very important part of our workshop. He became the "Moose Head Cook." Other people called him, "The Head Cook." He really, really loved it. We complimented him. He was so proud of himself. He would split firewood and kept the fire going under that moose head. He began talking to people. When we were eating in the evening, he was talking to everybody about cooking the moose head. He was empowered.

PUTTING THE VISION INTO PRACTICE

There were many changes in our community soon after the workshops. The main change was that it gave our people a purpose. The purpose was to get out of bed, to be able to go to work. It really helped, and what happened was that that the whole community began to sober up. We actually took a count—eighty-five per cent of community was sober. It was unreal—the difference in the people. When you give them a purpose, some hope for the future, and provide them with the services needed to sustain themselves, it is amazing what can happen and where you can go as a community.

Empowering people through building on their strengths is important. After the community development workshop, we knew that this was what we needed to do. We needed to empower the people to make their own choices. That's what happened. People started making their own choices, and they were healthy choices. They would ask themselves: "Shall I go to this workshop or not? What's my goal for today? What's my purpose for today? I need to get involved." People started participating in community activities and coming to meetings.

Another thing that we realized was that the administration needed more transparency. We needed transparency so that we could build more trust. And that's what we did. My father was the chief at that time, and there were four council members. The leadership of the day said, "What we need to do is to allow the people to come in and help us to make the decisions for our community, the healthy choices for our community to move forward." So that's what we did; we allowed them to come to the decision-making meetings. They provided advice for chief and council to make decisions for the community. We didn't shut anybody out.

Sometimes in those meetings, people would talk. They knew they didn't want to drink any more. One man looked at somebody in the meeting, a man who had bought a bottle and sold it to him to make money. He said, "I don't like what you did; you sold me a bottle to make money. Now I owe you a bunch of money and I don't have any money to buy groceries." They talked respectfully to each other. At the end, the man who sold the liquor promised, "I won't do that again to you. That's my promise." And that's what happened after the community development workshops.

We built an administration building. We had all agreed that was our priority. It was the first project on which we all agreed. So to do that, we had to install the septic lines and put in water and sewer into every house on the reserve. We needed to do that first because we needed water and sewer for the administration building anyway and because it had been one of the things mentioned in the visioning exercise. The next year, we started on the administration building. One of the things we did, based on the traditional knowledge of the Elders of the day, was to pour the foundation and let it sit for a year. Then the next year, they completely leveled everything out before building the building. This was the first seed that had come to fruition from the grass-roots community input during the community development workshop.

Today, we still don't have a community garden, but we do have a hydro plant that provides electricity for our community, and we are negotiating to sell electricity to the Yukon Territory. We are hoping to build greenhouses, using the heat from our hydro plant.

We began using art therapy when working with community people. I was shocked that our people could even do art. The next thing I knew, out came such beautiful pictures. We come from a very artistic group of people; it is one of our talents that we were born with. However, we hadn't been paying much attention to massaging our strengths.

We got everybody to draw a picture of what they would like to see in the community, and they had to tell somebody about their picture. I asked my cousin to tell me about his picture. That's when I knew why he liked to work by himself. We had tried to hire him but he always said he didn't want to work, that he didn't like working with a whole bunch of people. What we found out was that this man was gifted with an artistic talent. Since he didn't want to be around crowds of people, we started making contracts with him. It was unreal what it did for that man. He was so empowered. He walked around the community smiling and happy. He wasn't angry anymore.

This is the kind of thing we needed to work on, the grass-roots people and their inborn talents. We needed to build on the strengths of the community people in order to move forward at a community and at a government level.

A CHANGE IN FOCUS FROM
COMMUNITY HEALING TO POLITICS

There were many other ways we made progress throughout the years. We moved forward on community building for a time. Unfortunately, the focus on community development and healing gave way to a focus on politics. The people got left behind.

There should have been a third workshop to develop a community plan *for the community by the community.* There was a proposal to do so, but unfortunately, the funding was not granted. We also needed a structural assessment; our new health-related positions were just starting up and needed to be integrated into the overall administration. This was not done either, because we began focusing on politics and land claims instead of the community development and healing plans that we had talked about and started to plan for.

One of the changes we made over the years was to stop calling the leader of our government our chief. That was an Indian Act title. We now call our government leader our *Spokesperson—* someone who speaks for the community, not someone who tells the community what to do.

But politics is tricky. When I first started as Spokesperson, I didn't even know that politics could be a transforming beast. I came up with that name for it because people that I had known so well all of a sudden turned into "something else." I don't really want to say that, but that's what happened to me.

It was hard to take at first. It still is sometimes. It's hard not to take things personally. But I've come to realize that what I call politics, the *beast,* is mostly negative thinking taking control. It's lack of self-esteem. It's lack of hope. It's not wanting to get up in the morning because there is nothing worthwhile to do. It's thinking that somebody else can only get something by taking it from me. If we can't make the pie bigger for all of us, I can only have more if somebody gets less.

It's another form of intergenerational violence and lateral violence; it's about getting things by force and manipulation, not by working together in the Tlingit way. In many ways, we're back where we were in 1985. There's lots of drinking again. And now drugs, too.

PROGRESS THAT WAS MADE

There has been progress. In 1993, we actually finished a constitution and started working under our clan system order of government. We created a constitution that fits our Tlingit ways. On the website for the Taku River Tlingit First Nation, there is a statement from the Elders Council, as follows:

A governing principle in the Constitution is that Our Elders show us that, to live as Tlingit, the life breath of our culture comes from each of us through our heart, mind, body and spirit. Therefore, as Tlingit, we have a spiritual, emotional, physical, and intellectual relationship with ourselves and all other life.

Our Constitution is based on our clans and on our traditional values. It outlines the decision-making process based on these ways. In 1985, the leadership of the day was called *chief and council* because in those days we worked under the Indian Act. After we changed our constitution in 1993, council members are called Leadership and the chief is called the Spokesperson.

In the very first meeting that I had as Spokesperson with our three nations, the Tahltan, the Kaskas and the Tlingits, we all had to make opening comments. I actually spoke a little bit more than the others did, because it was the very first meeting that I went to as the Spokesperson for the Taku River Tlingit First Nation. I told them that I didn't want to talk about borders. The use of borders is not our traditional way. We have always shared the use of the land and welcomed strangers, but strangers had to respect our land, our water and our people. I urged cooperation between our nations when structuring how we use the land.

We are developing a land use plan and are mapping the traditional territories for hunting, fishing and trapping. Located also on the maps are the ways the land is used by the animals, fish and birds in the area, as well as the locations of natural resources of water, ore and mineral deposits. This mapping project will be used for Treaty negotiations, which have not been settled yet.

We are also working with consultants from various government and university departments to bring back our Tlingit language, to develop a conservancy area, and to return the geological landmarks in the area to their original Tlingit names.

NEXT STEPS

To summarize, many good things have happened, but today the people feel left out again, as they did in 1985 before the community development workshop. When we changed the focus to politics from healing, the people began to lose hope for change. Many began to return to old habits and negative behaviours.

In 1985, the people of the day said that we needed to find a way to include the grassroots people in decisions for community healing. We still need to do that today. We tried to capture that concept into the constitution because they were the same as our Tlingit way.

We need to include everybody. That's what I heard in the workshops in 1985. That is what I am still hearing. I, as Spokesperson, have started to include community members again and bring them in, so that we can make decisions for the community by the community. That's what it's all about. If people don't have input into how the community is going to be shaped, then we will have trouble later on. We learned that from our own experience. Leaving people out, that was never our way.

I am attempting to integrate traditional knowledge, our spiritual dimension, with the managing of all our projects. Sometimes this goes against government regulations and their ways of doing things. It is important for all those in the decision-making process to understand this spiritual aspect of our culture. Managing projects utilizing the spiritual dimension involves:

▶ Seeking advice from the Elders

▶ Planning based in traditional knowledge and family traditions

▶ Community planning by the community for the community

▶ Consultation with community members, community departments and government

▶ Empowerment of individuals in community, using their inborn skills and talents

▶ People making their own healthy choices and implementing them

▶ Emphasis on knowledge, skills, and best practices

▶ Building capacity, based on the strengths of the community

▶ Transparency of the decision-making process

▶ Interdependency, people working together to make community choices

▶ Interdependency with government, building partnerships, not dependency

▶ Using traditional ways of healing

▶ Using art as therapy to provide insight into a person's emotional/spiritual state

These are the kinds of things we are working on—our focus is the grassroots people and their inborn talents and how we can build on that strength to move forward to heal as a community. And we learned that planning is the most important part of any project for community healing.

My goal now is to find the money and build community support to have another community development workshop like we had in 1985. Thirty years is a long time to go without renewing our vision and goals for our community and our nation. A lot of good things have happened. But bad things have happened, too. The world has changed around us. We can't ignore that. If we don't adjust and make our own choices that respect our Tlingit heritage and traditions, we will have somebody else's choices forced on us.

It won't be easy. But it will be even harder to deal with the results if we do nothing. If we start, we will find the resources we need, just as we did in 1985. We have to challenge ourselves and each other.

I also want to accept the challenge given to us by the Truth and Reconciliation Commission in its ninety-four recommendations. I believe that is our road map to a better future for our community and for our relationships with our non-Tlingit neighbours in Atlin and the rest of Canada. We can't achieve all ninety-four recommendations at once. But we can work together to choose three, or four, or five priorities to work on for the next ten years or so; then it will be time again for another community development initiative.

REVIEW OF THE COMMUNITY VISIONING PROJECT

In reviewing the two parts of the Taku River Tlingit's community development story, some important lessons can be learned. These are:

▶ The importance of an overall Community Visioning Project, based on how community members would like to see their community

▶ Guidelines for decision-making based in transcultural values, meshing old and new ways of doing things

▶ The importance of a flexible blueprint for implementing the plan, subject to change as needed and as agreed on by others on the planning team

▶ The importance of teamwork, everyone being on the same page and following the same guidelines

▶ The importance of clear communication between funders and band administrators

▶ The importance of communicating with outside stakeholders about the community healing plan

▶ The importance of clear communication between members of the planning team and between the planning team and community members

▶ The importance involving community members in band activities as much as feasible

▶ The importance of having a personal healing component with ongoing follow-up programs and training in place.

And, as Spokesperson Gordon has said, "Everyone needs hope for the future and a reason to get up in the morning."

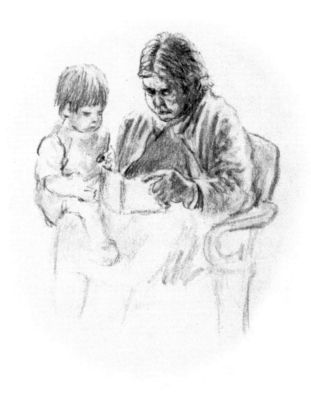

PART TWO

COMMUNITY HEALING CIRCLES

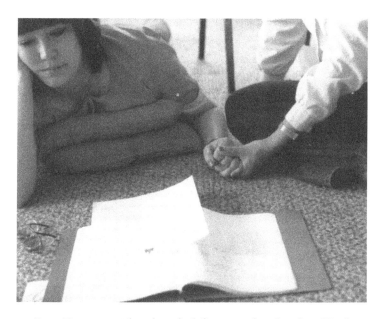

Part Two provides detailed formats for the five Healing Circles that make up the Transcultural Healing Model. Italicized words are to be read to the group. Non-italicized are instructions for the facilitator.

A Morning Prayer for The Healing Circles

Among my people we cannot come together like this without firstly expressing acknowledgement and respect for the Creator.

We come to you humbly, Creator. We give thanks for another day extended to us so that we can enjoy your compassion and goodness in life.

We give thanks for all the plant life, the animals in the woodlands, the fishes in the waters, for all the fowl and birds in the sky. In the universe we give thanks for all the stars and the planets, the moon and the sun. How can we feel superior to all living things? For we are all one. They, too, have a mission to accomplish. You have made each and every one of us unique and special.

We give thanks for each and every one here. May we learn from one another. Bless and keep our families that we left behind, our friends and relatives, too.

We also give thanks for our facilitators,* Geneva and Wilda. Give us understanding and guidance so we can appreciate everything in life that we take so much for granted. Help to open our eyes and our hearts to see the goodness and love that you, Creator, have given us. Help us to live and walk the right path that leads us to you.

Marlene Lightning

Elder

Samson Cree Nation

*Facilitators: change name(s) as appropriate

CHAPTER 8

PERSONAL HEALING CIRCLE, LEVEL ONE: WHO AM I?

"Loving your Self is the beginning of wisdom."

WELCOME TO THE CIRCLE

▶ **Lighting of the Candle**

  › Invitation to join the circle—Ask people to join you and welcome them.

  › Lighting the candle—*I am lighting this candle to mark the beginning of a healing journey for some of you and a continuation of the journey for others. We will light it each morning and put it out each evening, using it to mark our days in this Healing Circle. Since the beginning of time, man has needed fire, to warm, to cook food, to protect, to comfort. It can have many meanings for you as the week goes on. Right now, pretend that we are all sitting around a campfire.*

▶ **Inspirational Reading**: "New Warriors" by Chief Dan George

  There is a longing in the heart of my people

To reach out and grasp
That which is needed
For our survival.
There is a longing
Among the young of my nation
To secure for themselves
And their people
The skills that will provide them
With a sense of worth and of purpose.
They will be our new warriors.
Their training will be much longer
And more demanding
Than it was in olden days.
Long years of study
Will demand more determination;
Separation from home and family
Will demand endurance.
But they will emerge with their hands
Held forward...
To grasp the place in society
That is rightly ours.

Chief Dan George, 1982, p. 91

INTRODUCTION OF GROUP MEMBERS

▶ **Circle go-round.** *You will be asked many times in this series of Healing Circles to answer the question, "Who am I?" For now, tell us your name and something interesting* *about yourself that most people here do not know. Who will volunteer to go first? Then we will go around the circle to the left, each person taking a turn.*

▶ In this way, right at the beginning, everyone says something and the ice is broken about speaking in the group. You, the facilitator, can share as well, so that participants will begin to see that you are one of them as well as the facilitator.

INTRODUCTION TO THE PERSONAL HEALING CIRCLE, LEVEL ONE

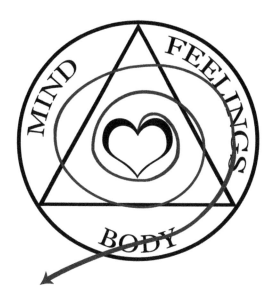

Figure 12 "All of Me in Balance"

▶ *The figure, "All of Me," stands for a whole person, complete and in balance. People have different aspects of themselves.*

To work on your healing, attention must be paid to all these parts: body, mind, feelings. Every part of you has needs that must be fed. The body needs food, clothing, shelter, etc. The mind needs to learn, to be challenged. You must listen to your feelings because they tell you how you feel about what is happening to you—whether you are happy, sad, mad, afraid, etc.

▶ *However, there is another very important part of you—and of all of us—that is invisible and often ignored. Within your center lies a Spirit, an Inner Self, who is a wise, knowing guide. The Spirit part of you is positive and is always there, no matter what has happened to you in the past, although sometimes this Inner Self is buried beneath a lot of hurt and pain. In this healing workshop, you will get a glimpse of your Inner Self/Spirit.*

GOALS OF THE CIRCLE

▶ Review the goals. These should be posted already on the wall.

> ➤ To begin to answer the question, "Who am I?"

> ➤ To identify what you need in order to take care of all aspects of your Self

> ➤ To discover and work with your Inner Self/Spirit

> ➤ To learn some tools for continuing your personal healing

> ➤ To experience the group as a comfortable, safe and healing community.

▶ *Do you have any questions, additions or comments?*

HOUSEKEEPING ITEMS

▶ Reach agreement as to:

- › Hours of work

- › Meals

- › Coffee breaks: morning & afternoon, when appropriate

- › Notes: Do not take notes; everything that is put on flip charts will be duplicated for you.

- › Calls: Will be held until break, unless there is an emergency.

... BREAK ...

ON FEARS

▶ Ask participants to open their journals and to finish the following statement: *"In this Healing Circle, I am afraid that..."* *Allow all your fears to come up. Be honest; don't censor anything. You will have a choice about which ones you share.*

▶ Allow time. *Now look at all your fears. Which one is your greatest fear? Put a check by it. What is the next greatest fear? Put two checks by it.*

▶ *If you are feeling brave, share your biggest fear with the rest of us; if not, choose one that you are comfortable sharing.*

▶ *Who will volunteer to go first, sharing your greatest fear or one you are comfortable sharing? Please make a complete sentence, starting with "I am afraid that..."*

▶ Some fears will overlap, but only list them once. Some people will have to be probed a bit to identify the real fear behind the statement. Go around the circle so that each person in turn will share one fear. List fears exactly as stated on the flip chart.

▶ *Does anyone else have a fear to add that is not on the flip chart?*

▶ When finished, give time for them to absorb what is on the flip chart. Usually group members are surprised that others have the same fears. Some typical fears are:

> I am afraid that I will cry.

> I am afraid of what I'll find out about me.

> I am afraid that I may get hurt.

> I am afraid that I will be judged.

> I am afraid that I will be too shy to say anything.

> I am afraid that I may be angry and want to run away.

▶ *Look at these fears; what is your reaction to all the fears on the flip chart? Would you be surprised to know that all people, when coming together in a group for the first time, have these same fears—or versions of them? People get good at covering them up, putting on a mask and not being real.*

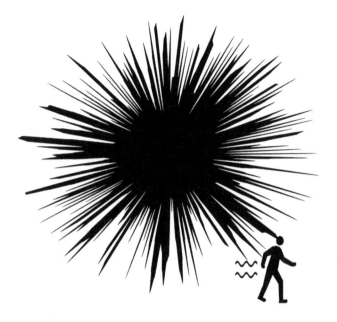

Figure 13 "Courage is born in the face of fear" — Rollo May

► *Fear can be like a huge monster. It keeps us trapped inside ourselves. When we run away from or try to avoid our FEAR, we give it our energy. It grows larger each time we run or avoid. If, however, we stop running, turn around and get acquainted, we take back our energy. We take back our energy and ourselves. We get bigger and the fear gets smaller.*

► *To face our fear is one of the most difficult things we have to do if we want to heal. In the process, however, is a great reward. We learn about ourselves and we start the healing process. Rollo May says, "Courage is born in the face of fear." Coeur is the French word for heart. It's okay to be afraid; facing our fears is an act of courage and healing.*

... BREAK ...

CREATING A SAFE PLACE TO EXPLORE THE QUESTION, "WHO AM I?"

▶ *Please look again on the list of our fears. If what you most fear happens in this Healing Circle, and it probably will, what do you need from the others in the circle so that you will feel safe enough to stop running and get acquainted with your particular fear?*

▶ **Circle go-round.** Ask a volunteer to share their fear, using an "I" statement, for example, "I am afraid that I will be laughed at." You could take this further by asking what word describes how they feel when they are laughed at. Then re-word the statement into a positive guideline: "I will not laugh at you; I will laugh with you."

▶ It is important that people's words be used as much as possible. However, encourage each person to start sentences with "I." Saying the word "I" encourages self-awareness, self-responsibility and direct talk, rather than indirect. It also focuses a person on their feelings rather than on words that are used to avoid feelings. Take all the time the group needs for the development of a safe place, because the members of the circle are building the foundation for later work if this is carefully done.

▶ **Circle go-round.** *Let's go around the circle, each of you giving one guideline that you need to feel safe.* List all of these on the flip chart with the heading Guidelines for Being in this Healing Circle. For example, typical ones are:

> › I will not repeat anything I have heard here.

> › I will not judge you.

> ➤ I will respect what you say.

> ➤ I will share my feelings.

> ➤ I will trust you. Although trust is learned through testing out these ways of being with each other and by learning to trust one's Self, as well.

> ➤ I will be on time.

> ➤ I will be responsible for myself. I can say yes or I can say no.

> ➤ I will ask for what I need.

> ➤ I will make "I" statements.

▶ *Is there anything else that should be added so that you can feel comfortable and safe in this circle?* Allow time for group to sit back and survey the entire list. This is hard work, so allow it to flow a bit.

▶ Check with the group. *Given the goals for our Healing Circle, will these guidelines help you to feel safe in exploring who you really are? If at any time, you are not sure what to do or how to be, check back with these guidelines. There is an interesting relationship between I WANT and I WILL. If I want to be listened to, then I need to promise to listen to others. In this way, your needs and the needs of the group are both honoured.*

▶ *Please write in your journals each night, answering the questions: What am I feeling? Have I been anxious or afraid today? What triggered it? What did I do about it? Has anything delighted me?*

... BREAK ...

GROUP WORK: BODY AWARENESS EXERCISES

▶ There are many awareness exercises to facilitate group members to become more comfortable with each other. Below are several possibilities; a few others are in the appendices. Structure these to the needs of the group.

Gingerbread Person

▶ *Turn to a blank page in your journal and choose a colour you like from the box of felt-tip pens. Close your eyes and draw an outline of yourself, starting at the top of your head and going all around, putting in an arm, a leg, another leg, another arm, and back to the top of your head. Keep your eyes closed at all times! Your drawing will end up looking a bit like a gingerbread cookie cutter.*

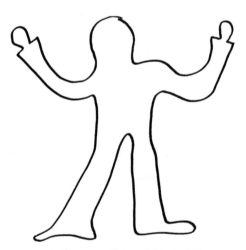

Figure 14 "Me and My Body"

▶ **Circle go-round.** As they share what they have drawn, there is usually much laughter and fun. Sometimes people see things that they did not intend to draw.

▶ **Body relaxation.** *Close your eyes, put both feet on the floor, take a deep breath and slowly let it out. Be aware of what is happening in your body. Where are you tense? Where are you hurting? What part of you is feeling happy or at ease? Using different colours, mark these feelings on your drawing.*

▶ *Find a partner; share your picture and what you were feeling. Did anything, any tension, hurts or pains, change as you became aware of them?*

▶ **If my body could speak.** *Close your eyes again, put both feet on the floor, take a deep breath and turn your awareness inward. Pretend that your eyes are searchlights turned inside. What is happening in your body? Check it out carefully. If your body could speak, what would it say to you? Write this message on your gingerbread person.*

▶ **Circle go-round.** *Share with the large group your gingerbread person and what you have become aware of during these exercises, using "I" statements.*

Healing Hands

▶ The following exercises often break down the self-consciousness of group members; they begin to become more comfortable with themselves and each other.

▶ *Everyone has energy in their body; in fact, we are energy bodies. Let's try this out a bit. Please stand and form a circle. Rub your hands together quickly and then pull them apart about two inches. What do you feel? Play a while with the energy in the middle of your hands; make a ball, roll it around. This feeling of magnetism is energy and can be used for healing yourself or others. When your body is hurting, you can give yourself comfort, ease pain and/or boost your energy level.*

▶ *Find a partner, repeat the hand rubbing and then hold your hands up to your partner's hands without touching. What do you feel? Play with this energy. Where is it strongest? Where are its seeming limits?*

▶ If the group seems receptive, have them place hands on a partner's neck or shoulders—with their permission, of course. What is each partner aware of?

... BREAK ...

▶ During the break, position blankets around the room so that each person has space around them. Place a pillow, legal-size paper and a box of felt-tips next to each blanket. Put a container with gold, silver and white pens in the middle of the room, easily accessible. Put on soft, slow music.

RELAXATION AND VISUALIZATION: A SPECIAL GIFT

▶ When group returns from the break: *We are going to go on a special journey—a total body relaxation, followed by visualization, something like having a dream. Find a spot in the room where you feel comfortable, and lie down on a blanket. Remove your shoes and glasses. Lie on your back with your legs straight and your arms parallel to your body. If you have back trouble, you might need a pillow under your knees, or you might want a blanket over you. Check to see if your body is comfortable. Any tight belts? Make any adjustments you need to be as comfortable as possible.*

▶ *Now, close your eyes and take a very deep breath to the count of four. Hold it. Let it out slowly, also to the count of four. As you are breathing in and breathing out, feel your body relaxing, letting go of the tensions of today...and of every day.*

▶ Repeat this at least three times, talking them quietly through the breathing in and breathing out count.

VISUALIZATION

Allow your body to return to normal. Imagine that you are outside on a sunny day. The breeze is blowing. You feel relaxed and very, very safe. Feel the sun's rays on the top of your head. You feel so good, so relaxed. As you are enjoying the warmth of the sun, you become aware that that a tiny window on the very top of your head is opening a little way so that the sun's rays can come in.

As the rays begin to warm the inside of your head, open your window a little wider. Allow the rays of the sun to penetrate each area of your head, relaxing, releasing tension, purifying. Feel your eyes relaxing; they do not need to see anything right now. Feel your jaw letting go, going slack. Feel your nose, your ears, and your brain—all relaxing. You have no need for thoughts right now. Let them float away on your next breath.

Now feel the warm rays of the sun flow down your neck and then out through both shoulders. Become aware of any tension, allowing the rays to surround the tension and breathe it away on your next breath. Feel the warmth flowing down both arms at the same time, then to your elbows, your wrists, into the palms of your hands and all the way to the tips of your little fingers. From your little finger, it flows into your next finger, the next, the next, and into your thumb. Your hands feel so light and tingly.

Allow the sun's rays to slowly return back up your arms to your neck. Feel the rays flowing down into your chest, into your lungs, into your heart, your liver and all your internal organs. They work so hard for you each day. See them working quietly; breathe away any tension that you find there.

Feel the warmth now flowing down to your waist, then to your pelvic area, down your legs to your knees, to your ankles and across the bottom of your feet. Feel the warm circling energy on the soles of your feet. Feel, really feel, your connection with Mother Earth. Allow the sun's healing rays to penetrate your toes, starting with your little toes first, then the next toe, the next, the next and then into the big toe.

The golden energy of the sun has given you a healing bath, from the top of your head to your toes. Become aware of your whole body. Is there any part of you that still feels in need of more of the healing rays? If so, take the rays there and give that area some tender loving care. **(Pause)**

You are now feeling so warm, relaxed and safe. Slowly gather up the golden rays and slowly return them back up your body and into your heart. Allow the sun's golden rays to completely fill and overflow your heart area. You feel complete, satisfied and whole.

Imagine that you are standing in the middle of your heart, surrounded by this golden warmth. You realize that an incredibly beautiful person is standing right beside you. As you look more closely, you realize that this person is radiating goodness, comfort and wisdom. This Being is your Inner Self/Spirit who knows everything about your life—who you are and why you are here. Take some time to have a conversation or to ask a question. **(Long pause)**

Soon it will be time to return to the Healing Circle from your inward journey. As you take your leave from this special Being, you are given a beautiful gift, something sacred that symbolizes who you really are. Accept the gift, giving thanks. Do not second-guess your gift; whatever image comes to you is the right one for this time.

Now it is time to return; you do not feel sorry to leave, as you now know that you have a special place inside of you and a wise Being to whom you can turn to any time you wish.

As I count to ten, slowly allow your awareness to return to this room. On the count of one, wiggle your toes; two, wiggle your fingers; three, four, move your shoulders. Five, six, take a deep breath; seven, move your legs; eight, move your arms; nine, take another deep breath, and ten, open your eyes.

Now very slowly and carefully, roll onto your side and sit up, staying in your quiet space. For now, do not say anything to your neighbours.

DRAWING THE GIFT YOU WERE GIVEN

▶ *Next to you are supplies: paper, felt-tip pens of all colours. Silver, gold pens and white pens are in the middle of the circle. Without thinking, draw a picture of the special gift that you were given. Don't worry; this is not an art contest. Fill the page; use bright colours; no pencils, no erasing or starting over. Mistakes are usually significant. Accept whatever happens without questioning.*

▶ Move softly around the room as they are doing this, checking to see that everyone is awake and drawing something. If, for some reason, someone did not connect with a gift, have them draw something—anything that comes to them, even if it is just a design. You can still work with whatever they draw.

▶ *After you finish your picture, be aware of any feelings or words that come to you. Write them in your journal or on the back of your picture.*

▶ *When everyone is finished, come back to the circle and place your drawing face-up and facing away from you, toward the group. It may be hard for you to do this, but it is an important moment, the beginning of opening up to the group and letting them see who you really are.*

▶ *How was the relaxation and dream trip? Are you okay? Who would be willing to share your awarenesses about the relaxation exercise? What was happening in your body? Where were you tense or hurting? Did anything change?*

▶ This is a general once-over; everyone doesn't have to share. You are just checking to see that everyone is okay with what has just been experienced.

▶ **Circle go-round.** *Who will start the circle and share something, anything you wish, about what happened in the dream trip? If you wish, you can share what gift you were given.*

▶ Allow time for each to share briefly what they were given, but at this time do not explore its meaning.

▶ *Tuck your pictures away for now; each of you will have time to work with your picture later.*

... BREAK ...

WORKING WITH MY SPIRIT/SELF

▶ This next work is literally the heart and soul of the entire healing model. You, the facilitator, should have studied and practised various techniques for facilitating deep-level work. Refresh your memory of the "Teaching Dream," outlined in the chapter on Healing Circles. Your job is to ask open-ended questions that pull awarenesses from each person as they work.

▶ *We will now be working with one person at a time, but in the circle. Who will volunteer to go first? You will know when it is time for you to do your circle work. Your heart will start to pound, and you will probably feel a bit anxious. This is the time to remember that courage is born in the face of fear. While a person is working, it is important for the circle people to listen carefully and be there for whomever is working. However, please do not interrupt or try to help out, like giving someone a tissue, until their circle work is completed.*

▶ It is important that people volunteer to work, that they are not selected to work. This is to allow someone's inner tension to build until they cannot help but work. That's when they are ready. Wait until someone volunteers to work.

▶ *Ready? First, please describe your picture, in general terms. What is it? What did you experience? How did it feel?*

▶ *Just listen to this explanation.*

▶ *Ask someone to hold your picture so you can see it from across the circle, and tell them why you chose them.*

► *Now, close your eyes and pretend that you didn't draw this picture. When you open your eyes, what is the first thing in the picture that you see?*

► If they say a mountain, ask them to describe the mountain as if the rest of the group had never seen a mountain. Ask a group member to jot down the words used to describe the mountain, i.e. very tall, solid, very old, here forever, cannot be worn down.

► *This picture is a representation of you—whether or not you can believe it at this time. So we are going to remind you of each word that you used to describe the mountain. Please use each word, one at a time, in a sentence, slowly and emphatically, as if you really mean it. For example, "I am a mountain." "I am very, very tall." Stay aware of your feelings as you say these words.*

► Ensure that they say these statements as if they mean them. If they cannot do this, have them repeat the sentences until they sound like statements, not questions. It may feel strange at first for them to be claiming these positive aspects of themselves. Probe a bit to see how it feels to be very tall or very old. This is the time to play. Trust your own intuition as to what would enable more awareness and acceptance of the words as being true. Have them stand and be the mountain. Maybe someone could gently push on the mountain to see if it is able to stand firm. Again, go with what feels right.

► Use the same procedure with any other significant object, person or colour in the picture. If they are stuck, ask the group to suggest some words that could be used to describe the picture. The person working can accept the suggestions or not, depending on what feels right.

▶ *Let's play with the picture. Turn it upside down, sideways ... do you see anything there that you didn't intend? Can you make any connections with the so-called mistake? Ask the others in the circle if they see anything when you turn your picture around.*

▶ Many interesting coincidences usually happen during this playtime. You will know when a gestalt is reached, when it *feels* finished for now. Ask for feedback statements from the group members about the person's work. How did the work touch hearts? What did they see in the picture? What did they experience as the person was working? This is not a time for advice, only sharing of other awarenesses and possibilities. What other group members see extends the awareness of the person working, as well as the awarenesses of the group members. Allow spontaneity to happen. Now that the major work of that person is complete, someone may want to give a hug or a blanket, whatever is appropriate in the moment.

▶ *What are you feeling right now? Do you feel finished? Please display your picture on the wall in a place that feels right and rejoin the circle.*

... BREAK ...

▶ *Whose heart is pounding now? Who is ready to work?*

▶ Repeat the steps. Take as much time with each person as needed until a gestalt is reached.

▶ This process may take several days. Work slowly and methodically, taking breaks after each person. Each morning, start the circle anew with a volunteer to offer an inspirational poem, prayer, smudge—whatever the group wants. This should be followed by a circle go-round, answering the question "Where am I?" These should be short statements, used by the facilitator for keeping track of what is happening to each person. Do not get drawn into working with these statements, as the pictures are the major work. Review the day ahead and begin the next segment of work.

▶ When all have worked: *Look again at your picture or symbol. Make a seven-syllable sentence that combines all (or most) of the good qualities that you discovered about yourself during your work time in the circle, i.e. "I am a beautiful lake." Or "I am a deep-rooted tree." Write it on your picture.*

▶ **Circle go-round.** *Share your sentence with us as if you really mean it.*

... BREAK ...

LEVELS OF MYSELF

▶ Have the drawing, "Levels of Myself", already on the flip chart. Say something like: *To ask the question, "Who am I?" begins a process of self-discovery. You discover that you are much more than you think you are. You have many levels; you are not a tiny person at all, but huge."*

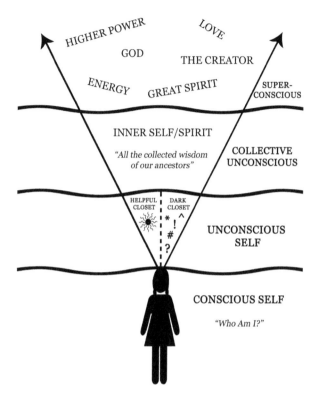

Figure 15 "Levels of My Self"

> The first level is the "Conscious Self." A person walking through life thinking that this is all there is: "I was born, I live, I work, and I will die someday, and that's all there is." Some people call this sleep-walking through life, or being on automatic pilot. However, we are much more than our everyday selves.

> The second level of ourselves is the "Unconscious Self." Our Unconscious stores two different kinds of memories. In a deep, dark closet, we store all the painful things that have ever happened to us, from the time

we were conceived. When things are too painful to remember, we shut the door on them and pretend that they don't exist. The closet can get too full. Nightmares usually come from this closet. Nightmares are important, because they tell us something that we need to be aware of in order to heal.

The other kind of memories stored in the Unconscious are helpful to us. All the good things that have ever happened to us are inside of us, as well as our bodily functions, the body's ability to heal itself, and our habits. Habits become unconscious and automatic, like driving a car or typing; we do not have to relearn them over and over.

If our dark closet gets too full, the force of unrecognized pain can cause the good side to stop functioning properly, and we will have a breakdown of some kind.

▸ *The third level is the "Collective Unconscious." A famous psychologist, Carl Jung, once claimed that all the collected wisdom of our ancestors is available to us— when we are ready to heal and to be healers in our community. This is a powerful concept. It says that culture and heritage are never really lost—just misplaced at times. Teaching Dreams often come from here. When we dream in bright, happy colours, we know that we are in our Collective Unconscious. It is at this level that people connect with each other. Have you ever said something at the same time as another person? Or been thinking about someone and the telephone rings? That is the Collective Unconscious at work. Inner Self/Spirit operates here as well.*

➤ *The fourth and final level is the "Super Conscious." It is called by many names. What is that something that gives life to our world and us? What is that Presence, that active force, which is larger than all? The Creator, Higher Power, the Great Spirit, God, Love, Universal Energy. Whatever we choose to call It, the truth is that the more we clear out and organize the Unconscious aspects of our dark closet, the more of our Inner Self/Spirit is available to us for living our everyday lives as a whole person.*

▶ *Any questions or comments? We have time for discussion.*

... BREAK ...

GETTING CLOSURE

▶ **Love Note to Your Self.** *In your journal, write a short love note to your Self, mentioning something positive that you have discovered about your Inner Self/Spirit.*

▶ **Circle go-round**. *Please share something positive about your Self that you have discovered during this Healing Circle. Also, share one thing that you will do differently when you go home.*

▶ **Appreciation of others**. *When we do deep inner work of the kind we have just completed, it is important that we let others know how we feel about them. Each of us will attach a flip chart sheet to our back, using masking tape. Walk around the room, writing something positive on each person's sheet, something that you have experienced during* *this Healing Circle. Sign your name. Make sure you also get a note from each person.*

▶ **Circle go-round**. *Take the sheet off your back and read each message; let the words sink in. Pick one that you like and share it with the group. When you are finished, choose a gift from the middle of the circle.*

... BREAK ...

CLOSING CIRCLE

▶ Standing, form a circle and read Chief Dan George's poem:

> *Keep a few embers from the fire*
> *that used to burn in your village.*
> *Someday go back so all can gather again*
> *and rekindle a new flame*
> *for a new life in a changed world.*

> - Chief Dan George, 1982, p. 60

▶ *What is one word that says what you are feeling right now?*

▶ *Who will put out the campfire?*

▶ Group hug

EVALUATION

▶ *Please fill out an evaluation form. Do not sign your name. All evaluations will be summarized; you will get a copy to add to your journal. See Appendix for a copy.*

NOTES

_____

_____

_____

_____

_____

_____

_____

_____

_____

_____

_____

_____

_____

_____

_____

_____

_____

_____

_____

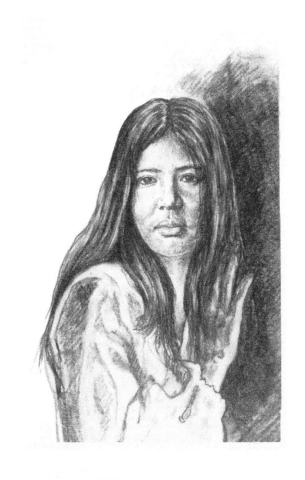

CHAPTER 9

PERSONAL HEALING CIRCLE, LEVEL TWO: WHO AM I?

"In letting go of my pain, I find the real me!"

WELCOME TO THE CIRCLE

▶ **Lighting of the Candle**

> Invitation to join the circle – *Welcome back to the Healing Circle.*

> Lighting the Candle – *The candle's flame symbolizes your Inner Spirit. The lighting of the candle symbolizes the beginning of another inward journey toward healing. Who will volunteer to light our flame for this circle?*

▶ **Inspirational Reading:** "A Child Learns"

When children live...
> *With hostility, they learn to fight.*
> *With ridicule, they learn to be shy*
> *With pity, they learn to feel sorry for themselves*
> *With shame, they learn to feel guilty*
> *With encouragement, they learn to be confident*

With tolerance, they learn to be patient
With gentle discipline, they learn boundaries
With praise, they learn to be appreciative
With approval, they learn to like themselves
With recognition, they learn to strive toward a goal
With fairness, they learn justice
With honesty, they learn truth
With security, they learn to have faith
With friendliness, they learn to be a friend
With acceptance, they learn to love
And to find love in this world.

– Author Unknown

INTRODUCTION OF GROUP MEMBERS

▶ **Circle go-round**. *Please answer the question again, "Who am I?" Tell us your name and something that you have changed, or tried to change, since the first Healing Circle.*

INTRODUCTION TO THE PERSONAL HEALING CIRCLE, LEVEL TWO

▶ Review with the group the model from Personal Healing, Level One. The figure "All of Me" should be on the flip chart before the session begins.

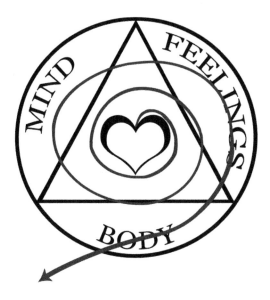

Figure 16 "All of Me In Balance"

▶ *This figure, "All of Me" is an ideal picture. It is important to get to know our Inner Self/Spirit and allow that knowing to help us in our healing. However, healing can be a long journey. As we saw in the first workshop, everything that has ever happened to us since we were conceived is buried in our Unconscious—in the deep dark closet. The negative things that happened to us, especially when we were too helpless to do anything about it, leave us with deeply buried feelings. For example, if a woman is pregnant and does not want her baby for whatever reason, what feelings might be left in the child?*

▶ Write across the figure "All of Me" the words suggested by circle members. Write these words in large letters all across the diagram.

▶ *Or what if the father is abusing a child's mother? What would the little child feel?*

▶ Continue to do this with various scenarios.

▶ *Eventually so many painful feelings get stored in the closet that a person no longer knows who they really are; the Inner Self/Spirit is covered over with powerful, painful feelings.*

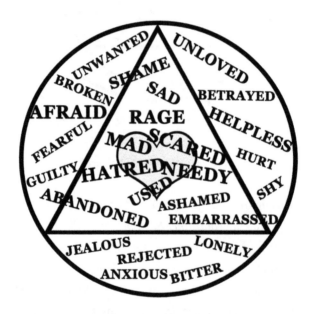

Figure 17 "Negative Feelings Block Inner Self/Spirit"

▶ *These negative feelings are in control of the person's behaviour; negative feelings usually cause negative behaviours. Therefore, in this circle, Personal Healing, Level Two, we will be working on what hurtful or negative feelings keep you from being who you really are. Take a few minutes and jot down in your journal some issues that are troubling you. Be as specific as possible. Then tuck them away for later.*

GOALS FOR THE PERSONAL HEALING CIRCLE, LEVEL TWO

▶ Review the goals. These should already be posted on the wall.

> ➤ To continue to work on positive self images and self-care

> ➤ To explore how your past continues to affect you now

> ➤ To work with a major issue from your past, releasing your feelings

> ➤ To learn how to use the Circle of Healing so you can be your own healer

> ➤ To continue to strengthen feelings of community within the group

> ➤ To get some rest and have some fun!

▶ *Do you have any questions, additions or comments?*

HOUSEKEEPING ITEMS

▶ Reach agreement as to:

> ➤ Hours of Work

> ➤ Meals

> ➤ Coffee breaks: morning & afternoon, when appropriate

> ➤ Notes: Do not take notes; everything that is put on flip charts will be duplicated for you.

> ➤ Calls: Will be held until break, unless there is an emergency.

REVIEW GUIDELINES FOR BEING SAFE IN THE WORKSHOP

▶ *In this Healing Circle, it is very important to feel safe. What was helpful for you in Level One? What do you need from the group in order to feel safe enough to work on the blocks that keep you from being who you really are?*

▶ List on flip chart—or ask a volunteer to do this.

▶ *These guidelines guide how we will be with each other in this circle. These guidelines are also healing ways of being which you can use with your family, friends and other community groups after the workshop is over.*

... BREAK ...

BE VERY AWARE OF YOUR BODY DURING THIS SESSION

▶ *Don't be surprised if your body starts doing things. Bodies reflect the emotions we feel. Every emotion has a motion. You may feel sleepy, tired, sick to your stomach, achy, twitchy. All are signs that something—some unresolved issue—is trying to get your attention! Pay attention and write about it in your journal.*

MINI-BREATHING EXERCISE & DRAWING OF SPECIAL PLACE

▶ *Most of the time, we are uptight and tense, especially when we do not want to feel the feelings we are experiencing, particularly if they are unpleasant. We hold our breath, tighten our shoulders and breathe shallowly to prevent our feelings from emerging. Yet, in order to heal, the opposite needs to happen. We need to learn to relax our bodies, breathe deeply and become aware of what is happening in us. Let's try it. Put your feet on the floor; shoulders back, take a deep breath. Let it out slowly. Feel the tension being released. Again, breathe in deeply; breathe out tension. Again.*

▶ *Remember the picture of your Spirit/Inner Self that you drew in the last workshop. That symbol represents who you really are at your core. Draw the symbol on the front of your journal and write a sentence, starting with "I am..."*

▶ **Circle go-round**: *Share your symbol and your sentence, i.e., "I am a mountain, tall, strong and eternal."*

▶ *When working with your feelings during this Healing Circle, remind yourself that your symbol is who you really are at the Spirit level, despite what you may be feeling in the moment. This circle is designed to bring up some of the negative memories that keep you from experiencing your Inner Self.*

... BREAK ...

CIRCLE OF HEALING

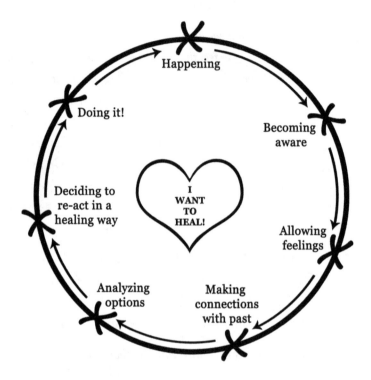

Figure 18 "Circle of Healing"

▶ *This figure is called "The Circle of Healing." It outlines the stages you will go through when you deal with your negative feelings and behaviours from the past. It shows you how you can change negative behaviour to positive choices and actions. Walk around the Healing Circle with me.*

    › ***A Happening.*** *Everything that happens to you can be used for your healing, especially if you feel strong emotions about the happening.*

> *Becoming Aware of the Happening.* As strange as it seems, when something "happens," you must first become aware of the happening. We often walk through life like zombies—unaware of what is happening around us. If we are unaware, we automatically repeat old, negative ways of dealing with our issues.

> *Allowing Your Feelings to Emerge.* After becoming aware that something is happening, you must allow your feelings to emerge fully and uncensored, no matter what they are. Allow them to come up; do not decide how you should be feeling or what others think you should be feeling. Feeling is not acting—that comes later.

> *Making Connections with Your Past.* When you allow your feelings to fully be expressed, only then will you begin to remember when you felt this same way before. In this way, you make a connection to the past. It is usually a painful happening that you have buried in your unconscious. This connection is called an "Aha!" It brings awareness from your past to the present.

> *Analyzing Your Options.* When you become aware of why you act in a certain way in similar situations, only then you can analyze your options for responding in a healthy way. Otherwise, you will keep responding automatically to the pain from your past.

> *Deciding to React in a Healing Way.* After looking at various ways to respond, choose a way to react that will be healing for you. Many people would like to stop here, with just thinking about it.

> ➤ **Doing It.** *The real test, of course, is to complete the process by an action; you must do it. When you do something, you no longer are a victim, because you have made a choice; you are part of a new happening.*

> ➤ *In this manner, step-by-step and event-by-event, you are regaining your personal power, the ability to say, "I am responsible for myself and for my actions." When you make choices and act upon them, you are no longer a victim of your past. You are a co-creator of your life.*

... BREAK ...

▶ During the break, position blankets around the room so that each person has space around them. Place a pillow, legal-size paper and a box of felt-tips next to each blanket. Put a container with gold, silver and white pens in the middle of the room, easily accessible. Put on soft, slow music.

RELAXATION AND VISUALIZATION: A GIFT OF HEALING

▶ *We are going to go on another dream trip. This will involve the same body relaxation that you did in the first Healing Circle. After, you will draw what you saw while on your dream trip.*

> ➤ *Find a spot in the room that feels comfortable. With shoes off, lie down on the blanket. For this exercise, you should lie on your back, with legs and arms parallel to your body. If you have back trouble, you might need a*

pillow under your knees. You might want a blanket over you, because a relaxation exercise always lowers your body temperature.

➤ *All settled? Check in with yourself to see if you are comfortable and that nothing is distracting you. A tight belt? Glasses? Make any adjustments you need in order to be present on this journey.*

➤ Give time for everyone to settle.

➤ *Close your eyes and take a very deep breath to the count of four. Let it out slowly, also to the count to four. As you are breathing in and breathing out, feel your body relaxing, letting go of the tensions and busyness of everyday life, letting go of any tension or fear. Welcome the relaxation as it oozes through you.*

➤ Repeat the count at least three times, talking them quietly through the breathing in and breathing out.

VISUALIZATION

Allow your body to return to normal. Imagine that you are outside on a sunny day. The breeze is blowing. You feel relaxed and very, very safe. Feel the sun's rays on the top of your head. You feel so good, so relaxed. As you are enjoying the warmth of the sun, you become aware that that a tiny window on the very top of your head is opening a little way so that the sun's rays can come in.

As the rays begin to warm the inside of your head, open your window a little wider. Allow the rays of the sun to penetrate each area of your head, relaxing, releasing tension, purifying. Feel your eyes relaxing; they do not need to see anything right now. Feel your jaw letting go, going slack. Feel your nose, your ears, and your brain—all relaxing. You have no need for thoughts right now. Let them float away on your next breath.

Now feel the warm rays of the sun flow down your neck and then out through both shoulders. Become aware of any tension, allowing the rays to surround the tension and breathe it away on your next breath. Feel the warmth flowing down both arms at the same time, then to your elbows, your wrists, into the palms of your hands and all the way to the tips of your little fingers. From your little finger, it flows into your next finger, the next, the next, and into your thumb. Your hands feel so light and tingly.

Allow the sun's rays to slowly return back up your arms to your neck. Feel the rays flowing down into your chest, into your lungs, into your heart, your liver and all your internal organs. They work so hard for you each day. See them working quietly; breathe away any tension that you find there.

Feel the warmth now flowing down to your waist, then to your pelvic area, down your legs to your knees, to your ankles and across the bottom of your feet. Feel the warm, circling energy on the soles of your feet. Feel, really feel, your connection with Mother Earth. Allow the sun's healing rays to penetrate your toes, starting with your little toes first, then the next toe, the next, the next and then into the big toe.

The golden energy of the sun has given you a healing bath, from the top of your head to your toes. Become aware of your whole body. Is there any part of you that still feels in need of more of the healing rays? If so, take the rays there and give that area some tender loving care. **(Pause)**

You are now feeling so warm, relaxed and safe. Slowly gather up the golden rays and slowly return them back up your body and into your heart. Allow the sun's golden rays to completely fill and overflow your heart area. You feel complete, satisfied and whole.

*You discover that your beautiful, special person is already there, waiting for you. You greet your Guide, thanking them for coming to visit you. Take time now for a conversation with your Inner Self/Spirit. (***Pause***)*

This Being tells you that they have another gift for you. This time, it is a "Gift of Healing." You are shown a picture of a very painful event that happened to you as a child. Go back in your mind to that time. See it very clearly, as if it is happening right now. Where are you? How old are you? What are you wearing? Who else is there? What is happening? What are you feeling? (**long pause**)

Now it is time to return from your inward journey to our Healing Circle. Thank your Spirit for your "Gift of Healing." Again, you do not feel sorry to leave this special place. You know now that you can return when you need to.

As I count to ten, slowly allow your awareness to return to this room. On the count of one, wiggle your toes; two, wiggle your fingers; three, four, move your shoulders. Five, six, take a deep breath; seven, move your legs; eight, move your arms; nine, take another deep breath, and ten, open your eyes.

Now very slowly and carefully, roll onto your side and sit up, staying in your quiet space. For now, do not say anything to your neighbours.

DRAWING THE GIFT OF HEALING

▶ *Next to you are supplies: paper, felt-tip pens of all colours, and in the middle of the circle are silver and gold pens. Please, without thinking or talking, draw a picture of the memory you were given. It was a painful happening long ago when you were a child. Allow yourself to feel your feelings. Fill the entire page with your drawing. Use colours, not pencils. Do not erase or start over. Mistakes are usually important. Accept whatever happens without questioning.*

Walk around softly, checking to ensure that everyone is awake and drawing something. It does not have to make sense to them at the time. It can look like a doodle or a scribble, but they should use colours. If a person cannot seem to connect with a childhood event, tell them to allow and draw any painful memory to emerge, even if it is a current happening. Give lots of time.

▶ **Circle go-round.** *When you are finished, come back to the Circle with your picture. Sit silently, aware of your feelings. Write them in your journal while you are waiting for the others to finish.*

▶ When the circle is complete:

> ➤ *How was the visualization for you? Is everyone okay?* Check to ensure. *Now, place your picture on the floor in front of you, facing the center. You might find this hard to do, but try it.*

> ➤ *Put this experience into one sentence saying, "In this Healing Circle, I am going to work on..."*

> ➤ When all have done this: *You were all brave to share openly what was a painful experience. Remember that courage is born in the face of fear. Remember too that we have all agreed to be non-judgmental and that whatever happens here is confidential. You are safe to work on your picture in this circle. Tuck your drawing away now until it is time for you to do your circle work.*

... BREAK ...

WORKING WITH MY PAIN

▶ Individual work in the circle with the facilitator. *Your body will tell you when you are ready to work in the circle, despite what your head might be telling you. Who is holding their breath or whose heart is racing?*

> › Wait for a volunteer. Do not choose someone and do not allow the group members to put someone on the spot. It is important that they choose to work when they are ready.

> › *Please hold your picture up and briefly describe what is happening in it.*

> › *Choose someone in the circle to hold your picture so you can look at it from a distance.*

> › Again, insist that they choose someone; do not allow a volunteer to help them.

> › *Close your eyes, take a deep breath, now open them. What do you see first?*

> › *Describe what you see and allow your feelings to be expressed.*

▶ From here on, you, as a facilitator, must use your intuition, experience and training. There are many ways to facilitate the release of deep feelings. It is important for the person who is working to express their feelings, not to talk about them. Use the gestalt technique for talking to the person who caused the pain as if it is happening right now. Use present tense and "I" statements, i.e., "You are hurting me. Stop!" or "I want you to love me" or "I hate what you are doing to me" or "I hate you!"

▶ The person working is encouraged to say whatever comes to mind, without censoring the words or the feelings. By venting real feelings in a safe place, the person then can make choices about what they may need/want to do later, outside the Healing Circle. Sometimes the release of feelings is enough to allow the healing to take place.

▶ Venting feelings can be facilitated by hitting a chair with a pillow or something similar. I had soft, stuffed dolls, one female and one male. They were used, and abused, a lot during these sessions. Feelings of hurt, anger and rage were visited upon them. They become tangible representations of whoever had caused the pain in childhood; they also can be a stand-in for a current spouse, parent or child.

▶ Emphasize and encourage the expression of feelings by asking them to speak louder or to say it again, and again, as if they mean it. Work until a resolution of some kind occurs, a gestalt.

▶ The group members may want to give hugs or wrap the person in a blanket—whatever fits with the work just completed. This comfort should only be given after the gestalt is reached; if given during the work, it distorts the process.

▶ When you sense the person working has completed what was needed, for now, give the circle members an opportunity to give feedback on what they saw/felt, but without giving advice. Keep the focus on the person who has just worked, not on similar stories from group members. This feedback is important. They will hear that they are not judged, that others empathize with or admire them. They will know that they are not alone.

▶ *Please tape your picture to the wall with masking tape and rejoin the circle.* Displaying the picture is also an important step in becoming more and more open, not hiding what happened, and now able to move on.

... BREAK ...

▶ Take a break after each person's work. The above is the main work of this Healing Circle—individual work with each person. Everyone's work is different. If someone is too inhibited to work with feelings, allow them to talk about their issue, but only after probing a bit. Some predictable issues are:

  › Being abused

  › Not being able to say "no"

  › Being abandoned

  › Seeing violence

  › Death of a loved one

  › Being taught not to cry

BEHAVIOURS RESULTING FROM "I LOVE ME" OR "I HATE ME"

▶ Pass out copies of the "Behaviors Resulting from Self Love or Self-Hate" figure.

▶ *Most people tend to turn their feelings either inward or outward. This is a way of looking at how negative feelings about yourself result in negative and destructive behaviour.*

*If your life stance is one of "I Hate Me," most of your be-
haviours will be negative. Some people believe that all destructive behaviour and all social problems come from a life
stance of "I Hate Me."*

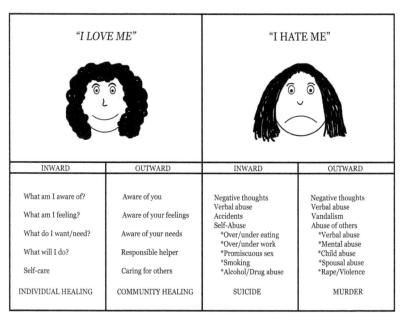

"I LOVE ME"		"I HATE ME"	
INWARD	OUTWARD	INWARD	OUTWARD
What am I aware of?	Aware of you	Negative thoughts	Negative thoughts
		Verbal abuse	Verbal abuse
What am I feeling?	Aware of your feelings	Accidents	Vandalism
		Self-Abuse	Abuse of others
What do I want/need?	Aware of your needs	*Over/under eating	*Verbal abuse
		*Over/under work	*Mental abuse
What will I do?	Responsible helper	*Promiscuous sex	*Child abuse
		*Smoking	*Spousal abuse
Self-care	Caring for others	*Alcohol/Drug abuse	*Rape/Violence
INDIVIDUAL HEALING	COMMUNITY HEALING	SUICIDE	MURDER

Figure 19 "Behaviours Resulting from Self-Love or Self-Hate"

▶ *Look at the "I Hate Me" person. Could this be you? If you
turn your hatred inward, it starts affecting your thoughts.
You may think that you are ugly or bad. The next level
resulting from "I Hate Me" is verbal abuse. Have you ever
sworn at yourself or have you ever said, "I'm so stupid!" If
you do not work to heal, your negative thoughts and negative behaviours usually increase over time. You can become
locked in a downward spiral of more and more serious negative behaviours. The end result could be that you say, "I
hate myself so much that I am going to kill myself."*

▶ On the other hand, "I Hate Me" turned outward follows the same progression, starting from thinking negative things about other people. Instead of thinking, "I am ugly," you may think, "You are ugly." Again, the "I Hate Me" life stance progresses to more and more serious behaviour until you may commit murder. You are really saying, "I hate myself so much that I'm going to kill you."

▶ As you can see, all Healing Circles or social programs designed to help people must deal with how people feel about themselves. Do you have any comments or questions about the life stance of "I Hate Me?"

... BREAK ...

▶ Let's look now at the "I Love Me" side. When you learn to love yourself, then you will begin to follow a healing progression, rather than a destructive one. The "I Love Me" life stance turned inward is the path toward healing and awareness. Checking in with your Inner Self will make you more aware of what you need. You are able to make healthy choices to fill your needs (body, mind, feelings, and spirit). This is taking good care of yourself. Doing this will lead to natural healing and the increasing growth of your whole Self.

▶ The "I Love Me" life stance turned outward makes you aware of other people, of their feelings and of their needs. You will now know how to become a responsible helper. Because you are in the process of healing, you know how to care for others and to assist them in their healing. Of course, you cannot do it for them! When you begin to heal, *your new way of being will bring about changes for other people in your life. As we heal together, the community begins to heal as well.*

▶ **Circle go-round**. *Do you have questions? Comments? How does this "I Hate Me / I Love Me" diagram apply to you? Do you make any personal connections? What will you do differently when you go home?*

... BREAK ...

GIVING VERBAL GIFTS

▶ **Circle go-round**. *You all have been very courageous to share your thoughts and feelings with each other. The more we can share with each other, the less we have to hide. The less we have to hide, the more energy we have to just get on with our healing!*

▶ *Sometimes we are not aware of how beautiful or brave we are until someone else sees us for who we really are. Who will volunteer to be the first to hear how others have seen you during this workshop? Everyone in the circle will say something positive about you that they have seen or experienced during the workshop, for example, "I see you as a courageous person," or "I see you as a beautiful butterfly, free." After your turn, you may choose a gift from the centre of the circle.*

▶ Repeat this process until everyone has been given verbal gifts and chosen a gift from the circle.

INSPIRATION TO HEAL COMES FROM MANY PLACES

Mother Teresa is quoted as saying,
There is a light in this world,
A healing Spirit more powerful than
Any darkness we may encounter.
We sometimes lose sight of this force when
There is suffering and too much pain.
Then suddenly, the Spirit will emerge
Through the lives of ordinary people
Who hear a call and answer
In extra-ordinary ways.

- Attenborough, **www.goodreads.com**

▶ *Chief Dan George has said…*

Love is something you and I must have.
We must have it because our Spirit feeds upon it.
We must have it because, without it, we become weak
and faint.
Without love, our self-esteem weakens.
Without love, our courage fails.
Without love, we can no longer look out confidently
At the world.
Instead, we turn inward
and begin to feed upon our own personalities;
Little by little we destroy ourselves.
You and I need the strength and joy
That comes from knowing that we are loved.
With it, we are creative.
With it, we march tirelessly.

With it, and with it alone,
We are able to sacrifice for others.

- Chief Dan George, 1994, p. 40.

CLOSING CIRCLE

▶ *Let's stand and form the circle. What is one word that says what you are feeling right now?*

▶ *Will one of you put out the flame?*

▶ Group hug.

WORKSHOP EVALUATION

▶ *Please fill out an evaluation form. Do not sign your name. All evaluations will be summarized; you will get a copy to add to your journal.* See Appendix for copy.

NOTES

_____

_____

_____

_____

_____

_____

_____

_____

_____

_____

_____

_____

_____

_____

_____

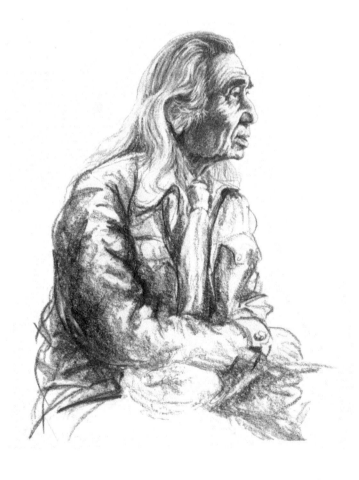

CHAPTER 10

INTERPERSONAL HEALING CIRCLE: YOU AND ME

"What's true for my healing is likely true for yours."

WELCOME TO THE CIRCLE

▶ **Lighting of the Candle**

› Invitation to join the circle: Interpersonal Healing

› *Lighting the candle for this Healing Circle symbolizes turning inward toward Self and turning outward toward another person who is important to you.*

▶ **Inspirational Reading:** "Kitche Manitou, A Prayer" by Arthur Solomon, a Nishnawbe Elder

> *Kitche Manitou,*
> *I send this prayer to you.*
> *I give thanks*
> *For the power*
> *And the beauty*
> *And the sacredness*
> *Of your Creation.*

I pray for my brothers and sisters;
I pray that they may learn to use your healing power
So that we may heal each other
And learn how to live in peace and harmony
As you intended.

- Songs for the People, p. 191

INTRODUCTION OF GROUP MEMBERS

▶ **Circle go-round**. *Please tell us your name and one personal change you have made since starting these Healing Circles.*

▶ *Choose a partner. Introduce yourself again, and tell your partner something positive that they don't know about you—a hobby, a skill, an interest.*

▶ Give about 10 minutes for this.

▶ **Circle go-round**. *Now, please introduce your partner to the circle, using what they have shared with you.*

INTRODUCTION TO THE INTERPERSONAL HEALING CIRCLE

▶ *Think back to our previous Personal Healing Workshops. The "All of Me" drawing reminded us that being healthy (whole, healed) involves a balance in mind, body, feelings and spirit. What we are feeling sends out an energy that other people can feel. When two people come together, the energy generated by their thoughts and feelings, whether these are positive or negative, affects the other person.*

▶ *As we discussed in Level Two of the Personal Healing Circle, how you feel about yourself determines how you affect other people and how you treat them, especially those who are close to you. It is quite simple: positive feelings about yourself create healthy relationships. Negative feelings about yourself create unhealthy relationships.*

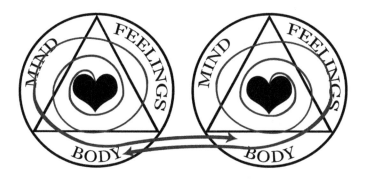

Figure 20 "You and Me: An Interpersonal Relationship"

▶ *Most of us are not aware of this connection and of our part in creating healthy or unhealthy relationships. Low self esteem, feelings of self-blame and unworthiness underlie all unhealthy relationships and ensure that negative relationships continue with our partners, our children and our extended family.*

▶ *To stop this unhealthy pattern is to STOP (literally) and take the time to reevaluate our way of being, learn how to change our behaviours and try out some new and positive ways of relating to the people in our lives.*

GOALS OF THE CIRCLE

▶ Review the goals. These should be posted already on the wall.

› To reinforce your awareness of who you are: a sacred being with body, mind, feelings and spirit

› To explore your way of relating to others, especially in terms of important relationships

› To become aware that you can change a relationship by changing your behaviour

› To practice healing ways of relating to others, including listening with an open heart

› To discuss how these healing ways can be applied to relationships at home and at work

› To continue to strengthen the bonds between group members, creating community

▶ *Do you have any questions, additions or comments?*

HOUSEKEEPING ITEMS

▶ Reach agreement as to:

› Hours of Work

› Meals

› Coffee breaks: morning & afternoon, when appropriate

› Notes: Do not take notes; everything that is put on flip charts will be duplicated for you.

➤ Calls: Will be held until break, unless there is an emergency.

... BREAK ...

REVIEW GUIDELINES FOR BEING SAFE IN THE WORKSHOP

▶ *What was helpful for you in Levels One and Two? Tell us what you need from the group to feel safe in this workshop, using "I" statements: for example, I do not want to be judged."*

▶ List on flip chart or ask for a volunteer.

▶ *Any additions? Questions? Comments? As mentioned before, these guidelines, or positive ways of being, help to create healthy relationships outside, as well as inside, these Healing Circles.*

GETTING ACQUAINTED AT A DEEPER LEVEL

▶ *You will find a journal under your chair. It is a good idea to write in it each night as the workshop progresses. What are your feelings, wonderments, ideas...? For now, please draw your Inner Self/Spirit symbol from the Personal Healing Workshop on the front of your journal, using bright colours.*

▶ *Choose a partner—someone you do not know very well— and find a spot in the room where you can talk freely. Share your symbol, being as open as possible, using "I am" state- ments. Please share as much as you are able; your partner is to listen carefully, asking open-ended questions to encourage you to share more deeply. When you both have finished, tell your partner what you saw in their symbol and how it felt to share.*

▶ Give about a half-hour for this exercise.

▶ **Circle go-round.** *Of what were you aware? What felt good? Did anything feel awkward or uncomfortable?*

▶ *The more open and honest we can be with each other without being judged, the less energy we expend pretending to be what we are not! When we are real, there is nothing to hide and a lot to gain from sharing at deep levels. Please show your symbol to the group and share a couple sentences about it—and you.*

... BREAK ...

ON LISTENING

▶ *We all need people; human relationships are fundamental to our survival in this life. Yet, how often have you stopped to wonder about what is involved in a good relationship? Have you ever asked yourself if you have what it takes to be a good partner? In this Healing Circle, we are going to look at relationships in several different ways, the first being your ability to be a good listener. Think about what the author of this poem is telling you.*

> *When I need you to listen to me*
> *And you give me advice,*
> *You have not done what I need.*

When I need you to listen to me
And you tell me why
I shouldn't feel the way I do,
You are trampling on my feelings.
When I need you to listen to me
And you feel that you have
to solve my problems
You have failed me, strange as that may seem.
Listen! All I need is for you to listen,
Not to talk, nor to do. Just hear me!
I can do for myself.
I may be discouraged or fearful,
But I am not helpless.
When you do something for me
that I should do for myself,
You strengthen my fear and dependency.
When you accept the simple fact
That I do feel what I feel,
Then I can quit trying to convince you
And I can begin to understand
What's behind my feelings.
When that's clear,
the answer is obvious.
I don't need advice;
My feelings make sense
When I understand what's behind them.
So, please listen; just hear me.
And, if you want to talk,

Wait a minute or two
And I will listen to you.

- Anonymous

▶ Group Discussion: *Did you really listen to what the author had to say? What did you hear?*

▶ Practice in Listening—about 15 minutes for each partner. Post guidelines for sharing on flip chart.

▶ *Think about some problem that you are having that you have not been able to solve. It can be about anything. Choose a partner and find a quiet place in the room. Share with your partner what has been bothering you. Allow your feelings to come as well. Do not censor them.*

▶ *Your partner will be practicing heartfelt listening. Listening with your heart means being fully present and open to the other person; your mind is not wandering somewhere else or planning what you will say in response. Listening with your heart means to be open to feeling what your partner is feeling. It means not judging what is being said, nor giving advice. When appropriate, a nod, a touch, a tissue may indicate that you are really hearing your partner. As the poem said, there is nothing more to do but to listen.*

▶ *Some guidelines for sharing are:*

  ➤ *Get comfortable, centered*

  ➤ *Make eye contact in whatever way is comfortable for you*

  ➤ *Use "I" statements*

  ➤ *Share sincerely*

> ➤ *Be aware of your body language*

> ➤ *Be aware of what you are feeling*

> ➤ *Remember that you are in charge of how specific to be*

▶ *When both of you have finished, tell your partner what it felt like to share heart space and, when finished, come back to the circle.*

▶ **Circle go-round.** *What awarenesses did you have while listening with your heart?*

... BREAK ...

BRAINSTORMING RELATIONSHIPS

▶ *Brainstorming means to jot down quickly all the words that come to mind without censoring, judging or being cautious. In your journal, finish this sentence: "ADULT relationships are..." with as many words as come to mind.*

▶ **Circle go-round.** Write the words on the flip chart under the heading "Relationships are..." Continue adding words until there are no more. It is usually effective to write the words all over the page, not in a neat column.

▶ *What are some of the words you used to describe adult relationships?*

▶ Take a few minutes for the group to absorb what is on the flip chart. *Do these words describe your relationships? Any other comments or awarenesses?*

... BREAK ...

LOOKING AT YOUR SIGNIFICANT RELATIONSHIP

▶ *Think of an important ADULT person in your life and write that person's name at the top of a blank page, just one person. Jot down all the words that come to mind, both positive and negative, without censoring anything. Your journal is a private space, so you can write whatever it is that you feel. When you are finished, sit quietly without talking and absorb what you have just written.*

▶ *Jot down any new awarenesses, feelings that you have about this relationship. When you are finished, write one sentence about how you would like this relationship to be different.*

▶ *Find a partner and share whatever you choose to share; remember the choice is yours.*

▶ **Circle go-round.** *Look at your list of words that describe your significant relationship. Using the same words, make "I statements," for example," I am controlling" or "I am demanding or "I am giving and caring." How does this feel? Did you make any discoveries?*

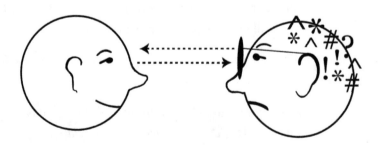

Figure 21 "Projection = Seeing in You What Really is in Me"

... BREAK ...

A WAY OF UNDERSTANDING RELATIONSHIPS*

▶ Draw the model on the flip chart prior to the session.

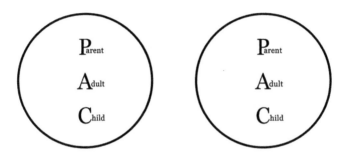

Figure 22 "Transactional Analysis Model"

– Berne, 1974, p. 30

▶ *As you already know, ADULT relationships can be very messy and complicated; they can also be wonderful. And we cannot get along without them. Humans need each other.*

▶ *Even though our relationships often are confusing and painful, we seldom stop to analyze or think about what is really going on. If you remember the Circle of Healing, you know that before we can change our behaviour, we must become aware of it.*

▶ *We are going to work with a Transactional model in order to see and understand what is happening in our relationships. It can show us how we are relating to others and how we can begin to change a relationship that is unhealthy. It may sound complicated at first, but you will see that it is actually very simple.*

▶ *According to the model, we all use three main ways of being when we are dealing with another person. Any time you say or do something, you are coming from one of these ways of being. These are called transactions. Transactions can be verbal or non-verbal, for instance, a wink, nod, and a smile are all non-verbal transactions. Some ways of acting promote healthy relationships; some create unhealthy ones.*

▶ *These main ways of acting in relationships are listed on the flip chart:*

  › *Acting like a Parent*

  › *Acting like an Adult*

  › *Acting like a Child*

▶ *When you were a child, you unconsciously learned to act in one of these main ways in order to meet your needs, to keep you out of trouble and/or to be safe. When you grew up, you probably continued your main way of coping with your world. Let us examine two of the ways of acting, the parent and the child, and the behaviours usually go with them.*

ACTING LIKE A PARENT

▶ *Acting like a Parent when dealing with another adult involves treating the other person like a child. Think of someone you know who always needs to be the Boss. What are the signs that someone is acting like a Parent?*

▶ List on flip chart. Some that should be included are:

- ➤ Controlling

- ➤ Criticizing

- ➤ Demanding

- ➤ Feeling self-important/ big ego

- ➤ Making decisions for others

- ➤ Taking care of others

- ➤ Being the authority

- ➤ Punishing

▶ *What do you feel when you are acting like a Parent?*

▶ Give time for responses.

▶ *What do you feel when someone else is acting like a Parent towards you?*

▶ *Any questions? Comments? Sometimes acting like a Parent is helpful, for example when taking care of an ill person. However, the focus of any Parenting of an Adult should always be toward promoting self-responsibility in the long run.*

ACTING LIKE A CHILD

▶ *Acting like a Child when dealing with another adult involves acting helpless and dependent. When you are acting like a Child, you need someone to act like a Parent. The two ways of being go together; one needs the other.*

▶ *Acting like a Child is done in two different ways: being a Pleaser or being a Rebeller. What are the signs that someone is acting like a Child?*

▶ List on flip chart. Some that should be included are listed below:

  › Is dependent, helpless

  › Has victim mentality

  › Has low self-esteem

  › Is always anxious to help

  › Is extremely careful, cautious, fearful

  › Is always angry

  › Rebels against authority, rules

  › Blames others; it's never their fault

  › Is sneaky, sly, manipulative

▶ *How do you feel when you are acting like a Child?*

▶ Give time for responses.

▶ *What do you feel when someone else is acting like a Child and wanting you to be a Parent?*

▶ *Do you have any questions, comments, observations about these ways of being?*

PARENT/CHILD ROLE PLAY

▶ *Find a partner and a space in the room where you are comfortable. One of you is to play being the Parent. Choose one of the ways of being that is on the flip chart, such as bossing, demanding. The other one will play the Child. Choose one of the ways of being a Child that is listed on the flip chart. Both of you are to interact with each other, staying in your roles as Parent and Child. It does not matter what the subject matter is; just go with your feelings and be aware of what your body, your voice and your heart are doing. Then switch roles. You will have about 20 minutes.*

▶ **Circle go-round**. What was happening in your body? In your feelings?

... BREAK ...

IDENTIFYING YOUR MAIN WAY OF BEING

▶ *Find a partner. Review with your partner both ways of being so that you are sure that you understand them. Share which is your main way of being—Parent or Child? If a Child, which Child? Pleaser or Rebeller? Do you change your way of being in certain situations? Why do you suppose this is?*

▶ Give time for them to process these ideas. Walk around the room, checking to see that they understand the two different ways of being.

▶ **Circle go-round**: *Come back to the circle. Please share what is your main way of being and why you may have adopted it.*

... BREAK ...

ANALYZING PARENT/CHILD RELATIONSHIPS

▶ *Let's look at the two figures on the flip chart. When you treat another adult person like a child, this is an unhealthy transaction. Why do you suppose this is so?*

▶ Draw a line from Parent to Child.

▶ *The destructive Parent/Child relationship appears in many forms: it is a power relationship, a one-down relationship, a victim and victimizer relationship.*

▶ *Even when you are helping or teaching another person, you are still acting like a Parent. It can be healthy as long as you are aware of what you are doing and why. The long-term goal of any helping or teaching relationship should always be toward growth, self-responsibility and independence. When you do something for another person that they could or should do for themselves, you are fostering dependency and child-like behaviour in the other person.*

▶ *When your way of being is as a Child, you will always be looking for a person to act like a Parent—someone to take care of you, to approve of you, to tell you what to do. Or you might be a Rebellious Child who always says, "No." You may blame others for everything that happens; you take no responsibility for your own behaviour. Sneaky, sly or manipulative behaviour belongs in the Child mode and is extremely destructive to relationships.*

▶ Draw a line back from Child to Parent in a different colour.

▶ *Every time a transaction is made from Parent to Child and Child back to Parent, this unhealthy relationship is strengthened. By responding in this way, whether you are Parent or Child, you are keeping a negative relationship going.*

▶ Questions for discussion: Write the following on the flip chart. What is the:

> ‣ Relationship between you and your adult family members?

> ‣ Relationship between your family and the community?

> ‣ Relationship between your community and the larger society?

> ‣ Relationship between your community and government?

▶ *Divide into four groups; choose one type of relationship listed on the flip chart. Apply this Parent/Child model to the types of relationship you chose. How does the model help you to understand what is happening in those relationships? Make a list of what you discover.*

▶ **Circle go-round.** Have each group report their findings and then open it up to a wider discussion of Parent/Child relationships.

▶ *Summary of Parent/Child Relationship: What is true for me and my significant relationship (micro level) is true for all other levels even up to the government (macro level).*

... BREAK ...

ACTING LIKE AN ADULT

▶ *Notice that there is another way of being that we have not discussed. The Adult way of being is when you are acting grown up. You are taking responsibility for yourself; you can say yes or no without guilt. Acting like an Adult can keep the balance between our Parent tendencies and our Child tendencies by making our own choices and allowing others to make their choices. It also involves being interdependent. What are the signs that someone is acting like an Adult when talking to another Adult?*

▶ List on flip chart. Some that should be included are:

  › Taking responsibility for self

  › Making decisions and choices for self

  › Talking to the Adult in others

  › Working cooperatively with others—interdependent

  › Listening to and respecting others

  › Admitting to and learning from mistakes

  › Working toward a balance of body, mind, feelings, spirit

  › Walking the talk

▶ Draw a line from Adult to Adult, using a different colour.

▶ *The goal of all relationships should be an Adult-to-Adult relationship. An Adult-to-Adult relationship is not a power relationship but an empowering relationship. It is an equal partnership, both sides responsible for themselves and respectful of the other. It is a healthy relationship, promoting and enabling growth for both partners. It is an interdependent one, each person able to be independent but working cooperatively toward the good of both.*

► *It is interesting that the more you know and love your Inner Self, the more you are able to be in an Adult-to-Adult relationship. The more you relate to others from your Spirit, the better you can see the other person and respect their Spirit. When your Spirit is relating to the other, your relationship becomes sacred, what some would call an "I-Thou" relationship.*

► *Do you have questions or comments on the Adult-to-Adult way of being?*

... BREAK ...

TO KNOW HOW YOU ARE ACTING, LISTEN TO YOUR WORDS

► *Count off by threes. Each group takes one way of being: PARENT, ADULT or CHILD. On flip chart paper, make a list of all the words or phrases a person might use if they are acting from this way of being. Add or draw the appropriate body language.*

► *When everyone is ready, tape your flip chart page to the wall and report on your findings.*

► **Circle go-round**. *What do you see? What are you aware of? Do you recognize yourself on any of these pages? Have you used these words? If so, how did it feel?*

► Pass out handout, "To Know How You're Acting, Listen to Your Words," asking different group members to read different sections of it.

▶ *This is a checklist to help you remember that by becoming aware of the words you use, you will know whether you are acting like a Parent, an Adult or a Child.*

TO KNOW HOW YOU'RE ACTING, LISTEN TO YOUR WORDS

ACTING LIKE A PARENT - THE AUTHORITY FIGURE
(INSTRUCTING, DECIDING, TELLING, TAKING CARE OF)

YOU SHOULD   YOU OUGHT   YOU MUST   YOU HAVE TO
LET ME TELL YOU   LISTEN TO ME!   I'M THE BOSS
DO WHAT I SAY   I KNOW BEST   DON'T DO THAT
WHEN WILL YOU GROW UP?   LET ME DO IT: YOU DON'T KNOW HOW
IF YOU DON'T DO WHAT I SAY, THEN I WILL...   WE WILL DO IT THIS WAY
DON'T DO WHAT I DO; DO WHAT I SAY!   I'M RIGHT! YOU'RE WRONG!
I'LL TAKE CARE OF IT/YOU   DO IT THE RIGHT WAY - MY WAY!

ACTING LIKE A CHILD - THE PLEASER
(DEPENDENT, CLINGING, WHINING, SUBSERVIENT, HELPLESS)

SO SORRY   PLEASE DO IT FOR ME   I'M MISUNDERSTOOD
YES, YES   I WON'T EVER DO IT AGAIN   I'M LONELY   TAKE CARE OF ME
I CAN'T DO IT   LET ME MAKE YOU HAPPY   I'LL BE QUIET
I'LL HELP YOU - IF YOU'LL LOVE ME   LOOK AT ME   SEE ME   I CAN'T
I'LL FIX IT, DON'T WORRY   I CAN'T   I'LL PAY FOR IT   DON'T BE ANGRY
LOVE ME   IS IT O.K.?   I'M UGLY   I'M NO GOOD   DID I DO IT RIGHT?

ACTING LIKE A CHILD - THE REBEL
(EXTREMELY INDEPENDENT, RAGING, BLAMING, ACCUSING, BULLYING, SNEAKY, MANIPULATING)

YOU MADE ME DO IT   I WON'T   YOU CAN'T MAKE ME DO IT! NO!
YOU'RE UGLY   YOU'RE NO GOOD   I'LL DO IT WHEN I FEEL LIKE IT
YOU'RE NOT MY BOSS   I'M TOO BUSY   "BUG OFF!"   I HATE YOU
MY WAY OR THE HIGHWAY   IT'S YOUR FAULT   I WANT IT RIGHT NOW!

ACTING LIKE AN ADULT - THE SELF-RESPONSIBLE GROWN-UP
(INTER-DEPENDENT, CARES FOR SELF AND OTHERS)

I WILL   I CHOOSE NOT TO   I WILL LISTEN TO YOU
I WON'T JUDGE YOU   WHAT DO YOU NEED/WANT?
I WON'T DO IT FOR YOU, BUT I WILL SHOW YOU HOW

▶ *Any comments? Questions?*

▶ Read: "I am my communication!"

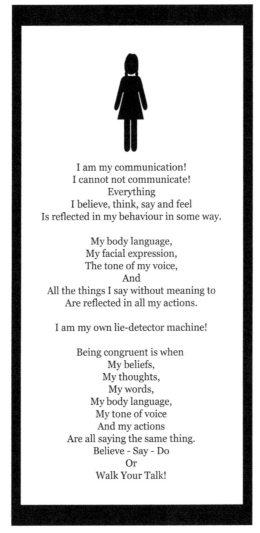

I am my communication!
I cannot not communicate!
Everything
I believe, think, say and feel
Is reflected in my behaviour in some way.

My body language,
My facial expression,
The tone of my voice,
And
All the things I say without meaning to
Are reflected in all my actions.

I am my own lie-detector machine!

Being congruent is when
My beliefs,
My thoughts,
My words,
My body language,
My tone of voice
And my actions
Are all saying the same thing.
Believe - Say - Do
Or
Walk Your Talk!

Adapted, Virginia Satir

Figure 23 "Being Congruent = Walking Your Talk"

... BREAK ...

HOW CAN YOU CHANGE YOUR WAY OF BEING?

▶ *The good news is that you can change your way of acting with another person.*

▶ Redraw the line from Parent to Child.

▶ *Whenever someone treats you like a Child and you, in turn, react like a Child, you strengthen that way of being with each other. It allows, even encourages, the other person to keep treating you like a Child.*

▶ Draw a dotted line back from Child to Parent.

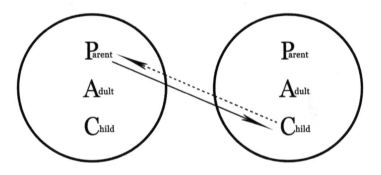

Figure 24 "Parent-Child Way of Acting"

– Berne, 1964, p. 30

▶ *If, however, you are aware of what is happening, you are able to choose to answer from your Adult. Take a deep breath; do not give your Child a chance to answer! Move your awareness up to your Adult. Speaking from your Adult, talk to the Adult in the other person. In this way, you are inviting them to move from the Parent mode to the Adult mode. If they respond back from their Adult, you have created a new kind of transaction, an Adult-to-Adult one. If they continue to answer from their Parent to your Child, take a deeper breath and keep responding from your Adult, using "I" statements, claiming ownership of your words and, therefore, of yourself.*

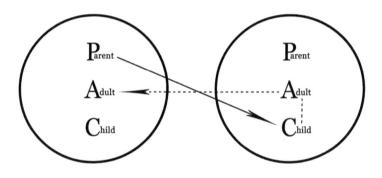

Figure 25 "Choosing to Act Like an Adult, Not as a Child."

– Berne, 1964, p. 31

▶ *Responding as an Adult, rather than as a Child, as expected, will probably come as a surprise, a bit of a shock, as it will interrupt the usual pattern. Parent behaviour cannot continue for a long time if it does not get a Child response. Sometimes, the other person's reaction will change from Parent to Child, but you must continue responding from your Adult to their Adult. Adult relationships are always equal and usually interdependent. No one is in charge; they help each other, as needed.*

▶ *Responding Adult to Adult, rather than as a Child, is a bit like changing your dance step in the middle of a dance.*

Something has changed; a new way of relating has a chance to emerge. This is not an easy process and may take many tries, but the more you feel good about yourself, the easier it is not to be caught in your Child or Parent. The first step always is to be AWARE of what is happening.

PRACTICE IN CHANGING MY WAY OF BEING

▶ *Find a partner, one person going first. The partner then repeats the above process, each helping the other. Draw a diagram of a recent Parent/Child transaction you have had. Were you the Parent or the Child? Briefly, what was said? How did you respond? How did that feel? What could you have done or said to turn the transaction into an Adult-to-Adult response? Draw it. What do you think could have happened?*

▶ Give at least a half-hour for this exercise, walking around to see if they are able to diagram the interaction.

▶ **Circle go-round.** *How was this exercise for you? What did you discover about your transactions?*

▶ *Any questions, comments, clarifications?*

GETTING CLOSURE

▶ Write these questions on the flip chart:

> ⟩ What was the most important thing you learned about yourself and your way of relating to others?

> ➤ How will you change your way of being?

> ➤ How will this change make a difference in your personal and community life?

▶ *In your journal, take some time to answer the questions on the flip chart.*

▶ **Circle go-round.** *What will you share about what you have just written in your journal?*

CLOSING CIRCLE

▶ **Circle go-round.** Verbal gifts. *The foundation of a good relationship is to have positive feelings about yourself and then you can have positive feelings about the other person. In Healing Circles like this, we see many kind acts toward each other, but seldom give positive feedback. Who will volunteer to be the first to receive some verbal gifts—positive ways that others in the circle see you?*

▶ *Each person in the circle will give you a one-sentence gift, using "I" statements. If you are being given gifts, open your heart and allow all the beautiful words to sink deeply into yourself. Don't respond; just listen and absorb. After everyone has said something, you may choose a gift as a remembrance of the Interpersonal Healing Circle. Each person will take a turn receiving gifts.*

▶ *Let's stand and form the circle. What is one word that says what you are feeling right now?*

▶ Read the poem, "On Lifetime Relationships."

> *Lifetime relationships teach you*
> *Lifetime lessons*   ·

That you must build upon
In order to have a solid foundation.
Your job
Is to accept the lesson,
Love the person
And put what you have learned
To use
In all your other relationships.

- Anonymous

▶ *Who will put out the candle for this Healing Circle?*

▶ Group hug/handshake

EVALUATION

▶ *Please fill out an evaluation form. Do not sign your name.*
All evaluations will be summarized; you will get a copy to
add to your journal. See Appendix for copy.

NOTES

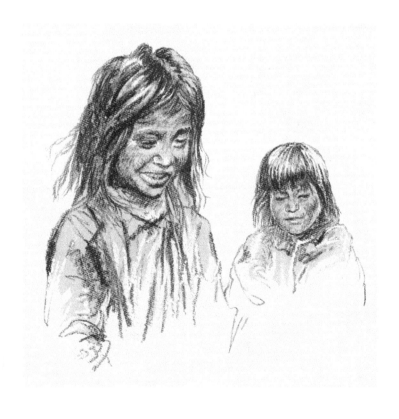

ſMALL GROUP HEALING CIRCLE: WHO ARE WE?

"The whole is greater than its parts."

WELCOME TO THE CIRCLE

► **Lighting of the Candle**

    ➤ Invitation to join the circle: Small Group Healing

    ➤ *The candle for this Healing Circle stands in place of a campfire. Humans have gathered together in groups since the beginning of time—for comfort, for safety, for survival. Today, you are here in a Healing Circle, with others, to look at your small work group, searching out what needs to be healed.*

► **Inspirational Reading:** *"All My Relations"* by Richard Wagamese

I've been considering the phrase "all my relations" for some time now. It's hugely important. It's our saving grace in the end. It points to the truth that we are all related, that we are all connected, that we all belong to each other. The most important word is "all." Not just those who look like me, sing like me, dance like me,

*speak like me, pray like me or behave like me. ALL my
relations. That means every person, just as it means
every rock, mineral, blade of grass, and creature. We
live because everything else does. If we were to choose
collectively to live that teaching, the energy of our
change of consciousness would heal each of us—and
heal the planet.*

- Embers by Richard Wagamese, 2016, Douglas and McIntyre.
Reprinted with permission from the publisher

INTRODUCTION OF GROUP MEMBERS

▶ **Circle go-round.** *In these Healing Circles, you have
been asked many times to answer the question, "Who
am I?" Take a minute to become aware of whether your
answer has changed over time. Has your sense of who
you are expanded? How so?*

▶ *Give us your name and anything you are willing to
share about how your self-awareness has changed.
After, tell us your job title.*

INTRODUCTION TO THE SMALL GROUP HEALING CIRCLE

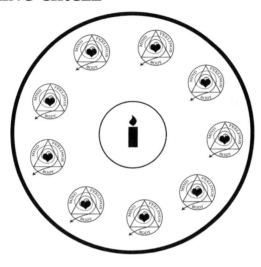

Figure 26 "You x Number of Members = Group"

▶ *So far, in this series of Healing Circles, you have spent time getting acquainted with yourself in several different ways. In Level One, you worked with a drawing of your Inner Self, your Spirit, that positive part of you that helps you on your healing journey. In Level Two, you let go of some of the pain from your past so that you could be more of what you really are. You also learned some ways to continue your healing journey on your own. In the Interpersonal workshop, you worked on ways to understand and heal your significant relationships. This Healing Circle will focus on what happens when you come together with others in a group to get some community work done.*

▶ *Groups are powerful environments. A group is made up of "You" (your body, mind, feelings, and spirit) times the number of other people in the group, with their bodies, minds, feelings, and spirits! Each of you bring into the group your individual history—all the happy, sad or tragic events from the past, all your hopes and dreams for the present and for the future. Imagine the bundle of energies and possibilities, positively and negatively, that are present in every group.*

▶ *It is no wonder then that when people come together as a group, certain things always begin to happen. Invisible, but powerful, bonds are created between all the members of the group. These bonds can be positive, healthy ones or negative, unhealthy ones. Group members often are not aware of these webs nor or of their part in creating and maintaining them.*

GOALS OF THE CIRCLE

▶ Review the goals. These should be posted already on the wall.

› To reinforce your sense of who you are, a sacred being with a body, mind, feelings and spirit

› To review how the group is organized to work together, what helps or hinders getting the job done in terms of its purpose, its style of leadership and of decision-making

› To learn more about each person's job and responsibilities

› To become a stronger team, fostering feelings of belonging and connectedness

› To apply what you have learned here to other groups in the community.

▶ *Do you have any questions, additions or comments?*

HOUSEKEEPING ITEMS

▶ Reach agreement as to:

› Hours of work

› Meals

› Coffee breaks: morning & afternoon, when appropriate

› Notes: Do not take notes; everything that is put on flip charts will be duplicated for you.

› Calls: Will be held until break, unless there is an emergency.

REVIEW GUIDELINES FOR BEING SAFE IN THE WORKSHOP

▶ Should be listed on flip chart

› *What was helpful for you in the other workshops? What do you need in order to be safe? Start the sentence with "I need…" Prior to the workshop, an agreement was made with the band that this workshop is truly a "confidential space." No one's job will be affected in any way for being honest and open in this Healing Circle.*

› *Any additions? Questions? Comments?*

… BREAK …

WHO AM I? WHO ARE WE AS A GROUP?

▶ During break, place a circle of paper on each seat. *On this circle, please draw the symbol that represents your most positive, powerful, wise self. This is not the time to be shy. In addition to your felt markers, there are gold, silver, and white ones.*

▶ Give time for this task.

▶ **Circle go-round.** *Introduce yourself to us, using "I" statements, for example, "I am a mountain. I am very ancient. I can't be worn down." If you cannot bring yourself to use "I" statements, then you can rephrase by saying, "My Spirit is like a mountain, tall, very old, etc."*

▶ *Working together, create a picture that represents your group/team, using all your symbols. In addition, you may use any of the materials that are here. When your group is finished, post the picture on the wall.*

▶ Do not make any other suggestions; give time for completion of the group picture. While they are working on the group picture, put these questions on the flip chart:

> ⟩ What are you feeling right now? Why?

> ⟩ How involved were you in its creation? Why?

> ⟩ Who seemed to take the lead? How were decisions made?

> ⟩ Overall, are you satisfied with the "finished product"?

> ⟩ Do you feel differently about the group now than before? Why?

▶ When people are finished: *Before we talk about what you, as a group, have just created, please answer these questions about the task you just finished. Jot down your answers in your journal. When you are finished, find a partner and discuss your answers. Remember to use "I" statements," not pronouncements. "I" statements take responsibility for your feelings and opinions.*

▶ **Circle go-round**. *Briefly, share your answers to the five questions. This is a time to listen to how others experienced this group work, not to debate any of their answers.*

▶ *What did you learn about working together as a team?*

▶ List these observations on flip chart or ask for a volunteer.

▶ *Add each of your job titles to your group symbol.*

▶ Give time for them to do this.

▶ *Look again at the group picture, made up of all your symbols and your job titles. Now what grabs your attention? Of what are you aware?*

▶ Allow time for speculation and musing.

▶ *Think about the vast stores of creative energy and wisdom that are within each member of this team. Positive energies build on each other and become more than any one person's individual contribution. When energies combine, something almost magical happens. Ideas, actions and solutions seem to come out of nowhere. This is synergy at work. The whole is greater than its parts. Of course, the opposite is also true. Negative energies build and magnify on other negative energies.*

... BREAK ...

HOW ARE YOU ORGANIZED AS A TEAM?

▶ *Every group or organization has some way of defining lines of authority and responsibility. Create a three-D organizational chart by arranging your chairs in order of lines of authority. What does your team look like? Is someone at the top? Is there a bottom? Or is there another way that you are organized to get your work done?*

▶ Give time for this.

▶ *Add your job title to your nametag and sit in your place in the organizational chart. Look around. How does this feel? Is this an accurate representation of your organization? Does anything need to be changed?*

▶ Give time for discussion and/or rearrangement of the chairs, until everyone is satisfied that it is accurate.

▶ *Let's look at what happens when a community member comes to the Band Office with a complaint or a request. Give me an example.*

▶ Write this complaint or request on the flip chart, i.e., "My next-door neighbours are partying all night."

▶ *To whom should they go with this complaint?* Tie a green string to that person's chair. *Where does the complaint go next?* Take the string and loop it to the next chair. *Where should the complaint go now? And then? And then? Who, if anybody, has the power to make a decision?*

▶ *Let's look again. In actuality, where does the complaint really go first?* Tie a red string to that person's chair and continue to follow where the complaint goes next, etc. *What usually happens next? Where does the complaint end up? Who, if anybody, makes a decision? Who takes action?*

▶ Repeat the process with other complaints or needs, as suggested by the group. Play with this, being aware of spontaneous happenings or comments, for example, the ball of string might be dropped accidentally. How does that relate to what actually happens in the office?

▶ Continue the discussion of the lines of authority and communication networks. How are they functioning and/or how should they be functioning? Allow time for discussion, comments and suggestions for improvement. Suggestions for improvement should be listed on the flip chart.

... BREAK ...

RE-VIEWING YOUR PLACE ON THE TEAM

▶ These questions should be on the flip chart:

  › What is your name and your job title

  › What do you do? What are your major responsibilities?

  › What do you enjoy about your job?

  › What do you find hard to do?

> ➤ How can members of this team help you to do a better job?

> ➤ What do you need to feel like a valued member of this team?

▶ *Using a page of flip chart paper and felt-tip markers, create a poster for your job by answering all these questions. Create a symbol that represents your job. You can use any of the materials—construction paper, string, etc. When you are finished, post your sheet on the back of your chair. Take about forty-five minutes to complete this. You may then start your coffee break while others are finishing.*

... BREAK ...

▶ **Group Processing.** *Please sit in the chair that represents your job or position in your office. This is an exercise in information gathering, not problem-solving at this point. When it is your turn, stand by your poster, explain your symbol and discuss your answers to the questions. When you are finished, tell the group that you are open to comments or questions. When asking questions or making comments, use open-ended questions and "I" statements.*

▶ Take breaks as needed.

▶ *These pages will be transcribed after the workshop so you can add them to your workshop journals as a reference for future teamwork.*

... BREAK ...

▶ During break, chairs should be formed in a circle again.

WORKING TOGETHER AS A TEAM

▶ Provide handout "Behaviours That Help or Hinder Working Together"

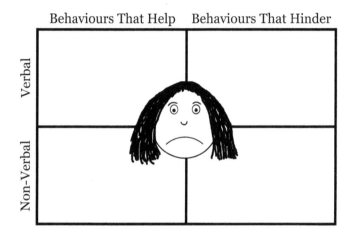

Behaviours That Help   Behaviours That Hinder

Verbal

Non-Verbal

Figure 27 "Behaviours That Help or Hinder Working Together As a Team"

▶ *When working in a group, your actions either promote group process or hinder it. You will have a few minutes to fill out this evaluation sheet. What have you seen in the workshop so far that has helped or hindered working together as a team? Do not add names, just behaviours.*

▶ Give time to do this.

▶ *Please form into two groups. Decide which group will take Helping or Hindering. Cut all the handouts in two, giving the Helping side to one group, the Hindering side to the other group. Each group is to make a collective list of behaviours that Help or Hinder the team's work. Add any additional ones you wish.*

▶ Give time for this. If the group is large, divide them into four groups, with two groups listing the non-verbal behaviours that Help and two groups listing the non-verbal behaviours that Hinder.

▶ **Group Processing.** *Choose a reporter from your group to present your findings to the rest of the team. Post your sheet on the wall and review it.*

▶ *Any additional comments? Observations? Awarenesses?*

... BREAK ...

▶ Provide handout "An Effective Group."

▶ *Group work professionals have been working on some of these teamwork issues for a long time. Here is a summary of some of their suggestions about what is involved in effective teamwork. We will go around the circle; each person can read one point and comment on it.*

AN EFFECTIVE GROUP

▶ Has a clear understanding of its purposes and goals

▶ Trusts each member; members feel free to share ideas, feelings and opinions

▶ Has feelings of belonging by all members (community)

► Has agreed-upon ways of doing things, including rituals and ceremonies

► Has good discussions, in which members clarify ideas by asking open-ended questions

► Makes decisions considering all viewpoints, reaching agreement and commitment

► Achieves a balance between getting the job done and meeting the emotional needs of its members

► Shares leadership

► Is okay with differences of opinion; members can agree to disagree

► Can talk about team problems, focusing on the issue, not attacking the person

► Works from a wholistic framework: body, mind, feelings & spirit

► Has fun and enjoys being together

- Adapted from Lippitt, Whitefield & Lewin

► *How does your list of helpful and hindering behaviours compare with this list? Would you add anything to your original list?*

► Give time for discussion.

... BREAK ...

CREATING POSITIVE GROUP WEBS

▶ *We all do our jobs better when we are seen and appreciated for what we do. As we have seen, teams work better when people are happy and feel that they are doing good work. We talked at the beginning about webs that are woven between people when they are together in a group. We are going to weave your web and make the invisible become visible. Who will volunteer to anchor the web?*

▶ Tie a yellow string around the volunteer's waist.

▶ *The anchor of the web will choose a person in the circle and, using their name, tell them something positive that you have noticed about them during this Healing Circle. For example, "Peter, I noticed that you are a good listener; you don't interrupt people when they are talking." The string is taken across the circle and around the waist of that person.*

▶ *The new person chooses someone else to compliment, until everyone in the circle has been looped in. The last person can hold the remaining ball of string in their hand or it can be tied off.*

▶ *Play with the web. You can stand, move around. Test the strength of the web. Make comments, share awarenesses of the web and of the team as you play. Have fun.*

... BREAK ...

CLOSING CIRCLE

▶ **Circle go-round**. *What is the most important learning from this workshop that you are taking home with you?*

▶ *Who will put out the flame for this Healing Circle?*

▶ Group hug, prayer or poem, whatever seems appropriate.

EVALUATION

▶ *Please fill out an evaluation form. Do not sign your name. All evaluations will be summarized; you will get a copy to add to your journal along with copies of flip chart work.* See Appendix for copy.

NOTES

CHAPTER 12

COMMUNITY HEALING CIRCLE: WHO ARE WE AS A COMMUNITY?

CHIEF, COUNCIL, STAFF

"Community comes from commune—to be one with."

WELCOME TO THE CIRCLE

► **Lighting of the Candle**

    › Invitation to join the Community Healing Circle

    › *Lighting of the Candle is symbolic of how Spirit has been bringing healing awareness to the members of this community Healing Circle, the leaders of our community. From here, it can continue to inspire the other individuals and groups in our community.*

► **Inspirational Reading:** *"We Can Change The World"* by Arthur Solomon

As Natives, we must involve ourselves in changing the world we live in;

*We begin this by changing ourselves. We are called to
care for ourselves and each other. We need to recognize
that we are children of God.
All effective change has to start with us. We can't change
other people; they have their right to be who they are.
We can help, but they are the ones who choose change. I
must look at myself.
Who am I? Am I happy? Am I in control of my life? Of
my destiny? Am I able to fix me?
I am called to care about my brothers and sisters. I am
called to be a beautiful person, a caring human being.
My teachers have been the earth, the fish, the animals,
the trees, the wind, etc. We all need to find good people,
for we have a need for nurturing relationships.*

- Solomon, 1992, p. 100

INTRODUCTIONS AND NEW AWARENESSES

▶ *After participating in the series of Healing Circles, you
may have had some new awarenesses about yourself.
Awarenesses come seemingly out of nowhere; a light bulb
turns on, and you may see or understand something in a
totally new way. Introduce yourself and share any awarenesses you may have had since the last circle, Small Group
Healing.*

INTRODUCTION TO THE COMMUNITY HEALING CIRCLE

► *This is the last Healing Circle in this series. The focus this week will be on the creation of a blueprint for the kind of community that you want to live in, a community that is a healing and nurturing place to be. In the inspirational reading, Arthur Solomon, Elder and Healer, wrote that we all need nurturing relationships in order to change the world or to change the community. How we can create a nurturing community is the goal of this Healing Circle.*

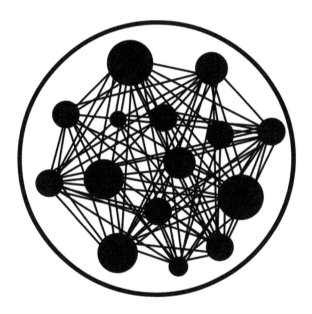

Figure 28 "The Reconnected Webs Between People and Groups = A Healing Community"

GOALS OF THE COMMUNITY CIRCLE

► Review the goals. These should be posted already on the wall.

- › To explore the meaning of community in general

- › To explore the relationship between your healing and community healing

- › To explore the question, "Who are we as a people— our shared values and beliefs?"

- › To create a Vision for the future of the community

- › To outline steps to implement the Community Vision, answering the questions:

  - » Where do we go from here?

  - » What are our guidelines for decision-making?

▶ *Do you have any questions, additions or comments?*

HOUSEKEEPING ITEMS

▶ Reach agreement as to:

- › Hours of work

- › Meals

- › Coffee breaks: morning & afternoon, when appropriate

- › Notes: Do not take notes; everything that is put on flip charts will be duplicated for you.

- › Calls: Will be held until break, unless there is an emergency.

REVIEW GUIDELINES FOR BEING SAFE IN THE WORKSHOP

▶ Ask for a volunteer to list on flip chart what needs/wants are identified.

▶ *What do you need from the group in order to feel safe enough to be real and honest? What was helpful for you in the other workshops? Again, it has been agreed that what is said here will not affect your job. You are free to be yourself.*

▶ Give time.

▶ *These now are guidelines for how you will be with each other in this workshop. The guidelines may seem simple or obvious. However, each guideline defines a healing way to be with people inside and outside the workshop, with your family, friends and in other groups.*

... BREAK ...

ON COMMUNITY

▶ **Circle go-round**. *When you think of the word "community," what is one word that comes to mind? Do not censor any thought or word.*

▶ Draw a large circle on the flip chart and write community definitions in the circle, but not in straight columns. Keep eliciting words until no one has any more.

▶ *When you look at this picture of community, what do you see? What are you feeling?*

▶ Give time for reflection and discussion.

▶ *Now, let us look again at this picture of community. Which words also describe your community?*

▶ Put a check mark by these words.

▶ *Who will add more words that describe your community? Pass marker to a volunteer. Again, do not censor any thoughts. Be real. Any other people want to add something to the word picture of your community?*

▶ Discussion. *What are you aware of now? What do you see? What are you feeling?*

▶ Don't rush these awarenesses and comments.

▶ *Some thoughts on the meaning of community. Community means different things to different people. To some people, a community is just a place on the map with houses, buildings and roads. To other people, a community is made up of invisible, but powerful, bonds that hold people and groups together. They believe that community is a group of people who share values, beliefs and ways of doing things.*

▶ *In a true community, these beliefs and ways of doing things come from the people themselves, not from some outside authority.*

▶ *When you were born into your family, you were also born into a community. You grew up and were formed and shaped by whatever was happening in your family and in your community—all the good and all the not so good. In Personal Healing, Level Two, you worked on some of your pain from your past.*

▶ *However, in these Healing Circles, you have learned that you do not have to be a victim of your past; you already have made choices to begin, or to continue, the process of healing yourself, your relationships and the small groups in which you are involved. The invisible bonds that connect you to others are being transformed from negative to positive ones.*

▶ *The good news is that as you and other community members heal, the community also is slowly being healed since it is made up of all of you. Therefore, the community not only has shaped you and your other community members, but you all have the opportunity to re-create your community into a place in which you want to live.*

▶ *How do you feel about these ideas? Are there other ideas or reflections you would like to add?*

... BREAK ...

MY IDEAL COMMUNITY

▶ Pass out legal-size paper and boxes of felt-tip markers. Gold, silver and white should be available as well.

▶ *We are now going to leave everything about your community behind, both positive and negative. You are going on a dream trip. Afterward, you will draw a picture of what you saw on this imaginary dream trip.*

▶ *Sit in your chair, feet on the floor, and take a deep breath, feeling yourself relax. Close your eyes and take another deep breath. Let it out slowly, allowing all your tension to melt away. Pretend your mind is a chalkboard. Watch yourself erasing all your thoughts and your busyness. Your mind is becoming totally blank; the slate is clean. Take several more deep breaths, letting go of any leftover tension.*

▶ *Now, imagine that you are living in a community that is very satisfying to you, a place where you feel secure, happy and fulfilled. You belong here. You are a part of a larger group. Visualize this community clearly: What does it look like? What is happening? See everything vividly—sights, sounds, colours, shapes.*

▶ *Become aware of the other community members, people who are also satisfied, happy and fulfilled. What are they doing? What activities are going on?*

▶ Allow some quiet time.

▶ *It is now time to return to this room. Take another deep breath, slowly open your eyes, and stay in your quiet space. Without talking, draw a picture of what you saw. Do not second-guess yourself. Draw the first images that come to your mind.*

▶ *This is not an art contest. Stick figures will do, but choose colours and shapes that vividly portray your ideal community. Take your time with this picture; do not rush. When you are finished with your picture, post it on the wall somewhere that feels good to you and wait quietly for the others to finish.*

... BREAK ...

▶ During break, tape four flip chart pages to the wall with the headings:

    ➤ THE INVISIBLE COMMUNITY

    ➤ THE VISIBLE COMMUNITY

    ➤ ACTIVITIES IN THE COMMUNITY

    ➤ MISCELLANEOUS

▶ **Group Processing.** *We need four volunteers to record on the flip chart sheets. Who would like to talk about your community first? Please stand by your picture and tell us about it, sharing everything you can remember. How were you feeling when you were visualizing it?*

▶ Give time for this sharing; ask open-ended questions if something is not clear.

▶ *Now, we are going to look again at your ideal community. We want to search for what is invisible. These will be recorded on the flip chart sheet under the label "Invisible Community." For instance, if there is a rainbow, tell us what a rainbow means to you, for example, getting rich, being loved, or being happy. Group members can make suggestions, but these suggestions should only be written down if it fits for you. This is your dream.*

▶ *The second part is easier. Name the things that are visible in your picture—people, places, buildings, machines, tools— everything that you can see. As they are identified by you or by a member of the group, they will be written on the flip chart sheet labeled "Visible Community."*

▶ *The third part is to identify what is happening in your picture. What are the people doing? Did you see children going to school? If so, what are they learning? People fishing? These will be listed under "Activities in the Community."*

▶ When something is talked about, but does not fall under one of the three main categories, write it down on the "Miscellaneous Info" sheet.

▶ *How are you feeling about this experience? Is there anything left unsaid?*

... BREAK ...

▶ Ask for another volunteer and continue doing this until all the pictures have been processed, taking breaks as needed. Breaks would be a good time to do some group physical exercise, stretching, energy work, etc.

... BREAK ...

WHAT DO YOU SEE?

▶ *There is an old song that says, "If you don't have a dream, how you gonna make that dream come true?" You have created powerful dream pictures of what your community could become. These visions come from the heart, the place of the Spirit. Each person's vision is important and has a place in the larger picture. When looking at the Visions as one picture, what do you see? What stands out to you? What is the complete picture? What are you feeling?*

▶ This is an important time in the workshop; do not rush people. Allow time for the whole picture to "sink in." As people make random comments, list them on the flip chart.

... BREAK ...

WHERE TO FROM HERE? — PRINCIPLES TO GUIDE DECISION-MAKING

▶ *How do you go about making the dream come true? Visionary dreaming gives you the overall direction for Community Healing, but there are many concrete decisions to be made when turning your vision into reality. On what basis will these decisions be made?*

▶ *Just as you created guidelines for being safe and comfortable in these Healing Circles, you need to outline the overall principles that will guide all your subsequent planning and decision-making. For example, when someone suggests a program for the community, but it goes against one of your basic principles, then that program should not be approved. Examples of principles: equality of all people, people-centered decision-making, culturally relevant programs.*

▶ *Break into groups of three and find a quiet corner. Make a list of the principles that need to guide the decision-making process. Write down whatever is suggested without challenge. After you have completed a list, discuss each item and come to an agreement as to whether or not this should be listed as a principle for all decision-making. Take as much time as you need. When you are finished, post your sheet on the wall.*

▶ **Group Processing**. Each group in turn reports their findings.

▶ *Can these be combined into one list? Can we come to a group consensus and make a final list?*

... BREAK ...

▶ *Here are principles that were developed by a community development specialist. Look them over and see how they compare with your list. What fits? What doesn't?*

COMMUNITY PLANNING PRINCIPLES

PRINCIPLES:

▶ Every person in a community is valuable and *has inherent worth and dignity.*

▶ *Self-determination* is a basic right and responsibility of individuals and groups, meaning the ability to make decisions individually and with others for the good of the group.

▶ Within each person are *the desire and ability,* to learn, grow and develop.

▶ Growth implies *positive development* in all aspects of one's self: Body, Mind, Feelings, and Spirit.

▶ Each individual has a unique contribution to make to the *life* of a community.

▶ Community change *happens* as individuals within it grow and change.

THEREFORE, COMMUNITY PLANNING WILL:

▶ Be concerned with the overall well-being of all community members

▶ Be concerned with facilitating growth by deliberate, conscious action and planning

▶ Integrate and use knowledge and expertise from all disciplines

▶ Work with community people in various combinations: individuals, one-to-one, small groups, inter-group and the community as a whole

▶ Be based in self-help and self-responsibility

▶ Be based in participation, involvement and cooperative action

▶ Work with self and/or community-identified issues, not pre-determined agendas

▶ Use conscious decision-making or general agreement, not majority win

▶ Emphasize process (people participation and cooperation) over a predetermined result

▶ Be long-term, not a crash program

Adapted from Dunham, 1970, 172-173.

▶ When the discussion is finished, end it with the following summary:

Community = self-made bonds between people

Community Development = processes and programs that facilitate positive self-made bonds

Community Healing = positive self-made bonds at all levels

WHERE TO FROM HERE? — NEXT STEPS

▶ *You have done a lot of work during this Healing Circle. You now have a Community Vision and have outlined the guidelines for decision-making when turning the Vision into reality. In the process, a lot of healing has already taken place.*

▶ *As a chief and council, what should happen next?*

▶ List all suggested possibilities on flip chart. Some possibilities could be:

▶ For chief and council:
  › To develop a plan for implementing the Community Vision

  › To assign individual roles, responsibilities

  › To continue to promote togetherness and team building among the staff

▶ For community members:
  › To share the chief and council's Vision

  › To provide an opportunity for them to be a part of planning for the future

  › To foster and strengthen the feeling of community

  › To offer the Healing Circles to all community members.

▶ *Which one should be first, second, third?*

▶ *Any questions? Comments? Dangling strings?*

CLOSING CIRCLE

▶ Close the Community Healing Circle by standing and joining hands.

▶ *In closing, who will read some advice from the late Richard Wagamese, an Indigenous Canadian writer and spiritual leader, on how to make a dream come true?*

> *"Don't focus on the dream, or it will always remain a dream. Instead, focus on the first action you can take to bring that dream a little closer. Then take it. Now focus on the next action, and take that. Each step brings the dream closer to becoming reality. Why? Our elders teach that the dream world and the real world operate on the same energy. You link them through the power of choice. Choose action and the dream moves ever closer to the real."*

> - *Embers by Richard Wagamese*, 2016, Douglas and McIntyre. Reprinted with permission from the publisher

▶ *What is one word to describe what Community Healing means to you?*

▶ *Who will put out the flame?*

▶ Hugs or handshakes.

EVALUATION

▶ *Please fill out an evaluation form. Do not sign your name. All evaluations will be summarized; you will get a copy to add to your journal, along with copies of the flip chart material.* See Appendix for copy .

This Community Healing Circle can be adapted to include other types of community groups.

NOTES

THE SUMMING UP

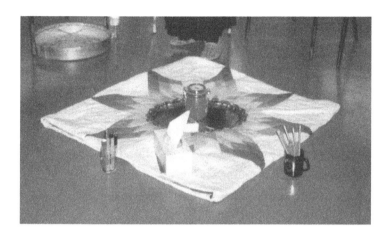

"Healing Circles bring hope to the hopeless."

In March of 2016, National Chief Perry Bellegarde, Assembly of First Nations, discussed the issue of teen suicides in Cross Lake, Manitoba. He said, "It's a bigger issue than just Cross Lake." He called for a huge intervention, a mental health national strategy to deal with the youth suicide. "Our young people need hope and inspiration," he said. They don't see that right now. We've got to make those key strategic interventions now. It's a life-and-death situation."

A month later, Dr. Laurence Kirmayer, director, Network for Aboriginal Mental Health Research, was quoted as saying that suicide can be seen as an idea that is talked about and modeled, an idea that can spread from person to person, almost like the spread of a virus. He thought that this was especially true in isolated Northern communities. He went on to say that human beings can cope *if they have hope*. However, if they have no reason to think that there can be a better tomorrow, then they are stuck between the past and the present, feeling that they have no options for the future.

Although these comments were made in response to the epidemic of teen suicides, they also apply to their communities as a whole, since despairing teenagers are a mirror reflection of the chaos, pain and hopelessness that is occurring in the broader community. The Community Healing Model outlined in this book offers a series of Healing Circles that are designed to bring hope and purpose to individuals and communities in crisis.

The model is a blending of transcultural approaches to healing. The philosophy of community development proposes that within each person is the desire and the ability to grow and develop, a force that moves individuals toward wholeness and health. Transpersonal psychologists talk about an Inner Self that guides the process of becoming who one is meant to be, and Indigenous spiritual Elders believe that all individuals have a Spirit that teaches and instructs, drawing individuals toward healing and wholeness.

In the words of the Elders, this Spirit has lain dormant for many, many years; individuals and communities have collapsed without this integrating spiritual force as their centre. When external services are provided to a community—more money, better houses, more programming, an improved infrastructure or even counselling services—without dealing with the underlying symptoms of community disorganization, all this external motivation will ultimately fail. Healing must come from within—from reconnecting with who one really is, the Inner Self/Spirit. All lasting motivation for individuals to change comes from this internal source, after which it can move outward, bringing changed behaviours within the family and the community.

For those uncomfortable with the words Spirit/Inner Self, the word *love* can be substituted. Whatever words are used, when individuals learn that they are more than a bundle of hurts and pains, that they are potentially beautiful, powerful and wise, their attitude toward themselves begins to change. They learn that they are worthy of love and respect. These positive changes in attitude enable a person to come to terms with the traumas of the past and to find hope and direction for the future. When this healing takes place in the midst of a Healing Circle, new, positive behaviours become the norm. Now a *healing virus* has been activated in the community because one person's change invites, sometimes impels, others to change also. There is a new dance in town.

The model involves five Healing Circles. They are:

▶ Personal Healing, Level One

▶ Personal Healing, Level Two

▶ Interpersonal Healing

▶ Small Group/Staff Development Healing

▶ Community Healing

Healing Circle exercises have been carefully designed to involve participants in their own healing. The healing principles used in the first circle, Personal Healing, are incorporated in all the subsequent Healing Circles. The basic question, "Who am I?" is asked and reinforced at all the levels of the healing model. Each time that question is asked and answered, an individual's awareness of self, and the manner in which they relate to others, is deepened and strengthened.

This transcultural approach does not negate cultural truths, as one cannot separate self from culture. To work with what it means to be *a human* is a safe and solid foundation on which to create healing relationships. The teaching of specific cultural beliefs and practices is not a part of this model, yet when members of the circle share their values and beliefs, culture is being acknowledged and respected. Cultural teachings can be a natural partner, given in conjunction with the Healing Circles.

THE BROADER ISSUE

The Truth and Reconciliation Commission has emphasized that a focus just on community healing is not enough, that healing is a Canada-wide responsibility. In March 2017, CBC reported Senator Murray Sinclair, head of the Truth and Reconciliation Commission, as saying that while government has been slow to respond to the ninety-four calls to action, it's up to society to take the actions that are needed.

In January 2017, Stan Chung, in Kelowna's *Daily Courier,* wrote that for true reconciliation to take place in Canadian society, it requires that non-Indigenous people experience a transformation in their own attitudes and actions. He asked, "How do we become allies to Indigenous people without re-committing colonization in a different guise?" The answer for him was for the non-Indigenous community to acknowledge, recognize, and explore the Other within.

Doug Heckbert, former training coordinator for Native Counselling Services of Alberta, stressed the importance of partnerships. He said, "To me, the word 'partnership' seems to be the right framework for discussions and actions related to the Indigenous communities. It means we must learn about the Indigenous experience, with all the joys and sorrows that go with it."

Reconciliation requires a partnership model to replace the colonial one. Colonialism is the exploitation and subjugation of a people by a larger power, whereas a relationship between partners is one of equality. In addition, equality requires an attitude change, a willingness to "see ourselves as others see us." In partnerships, both sides have power, each having something to give and something to get. In Transactional Analysis terms, this equality would be called an Adult-to-Adult relationship. For too long the colonial model has fostered an Adult-to-Child relationship.

The Community Healing Model described in this book evolved over a forty-year time span while facilitating individual and group psychotherapy. Planning and implementation of workshops was always conducted as a partnership between me and the Indigenous groups and organizations sponsoring them. The model was forged out of this transcultural milieu, both partners contributing to the final product. It certainly was a two-way street.

An example of this is how my working relationship with the late Wilda Louis, an Elder on the Samson Cree Nation, turned into a deep friendship. Wilda, as the Director of Social Programs, contracted with me to conduct residential Women's Therapy Groups. While attending the group, she discovered that she needed to work on some of her own issues. She requested to become my client in one-to-one therapy sessions.

Later, she organized a new program for the Samson Band called Community Wellness, again contracting with me to facilitate additional women's groups. Over time, as she learned about groups by attending all of the sessions with her own clients, she became my co-therapist, contributing valuable insights and suggestions for improvements. Through this process, we became good friends as well as working colleagues and partners. When I retired, she continued facilitating the groups, expanding them to include men's groups and one-to-one counselling. Her work was not a nine-to-five job. When she passed away in May 2017, there was a huge outpouring of love and appreciation at her wake and her funeral for all she had done for the people of the Samson Cree Nation. I will miss her greatly.

Canada-wide healing and reconciliation is a huge concept, a vast undertaking that will take many years to unfold. It is happening, but slowly, as Senator Sinclair has pointed out. Yet he is calling for action *now*. He said, "Actions speak louder than words. The reality is that we're really looking for action that shows leadership, that causes people to sit up and take notice and recognize that there is an important process underway here that they have to be part of." Senator Sinclair is proposing massive changes to the political and social structure of Canadian society, and he is also calling for the ordinary citizens to *take responsibility* and *to take action* toward the goal of reconciliation *now*.

Change, real and lasting change, is brought about through changes of the *heart and mind,* through person-to-person contact, through the realization that *the Other* is *Me.* Although most of us cannot bring about massive societal changes through our efforts, we can contribute to reconciliation by initiating many smaller projects across Canada.

This is the context in which *Community Healing: A Transcultural Model* was written. Its focus is on the implementation of the model in a specific community in crisis. Yet, if one dares to think Canada-wide, instead of just community-wide, then a broader dream is possible. The dream would involve:

▶ The establishment of a training centre, or institute, for Community Healing; this could be undertaken by a community college on one of the reserves and funded by a partnership of public and private monies.

▶ The training of healing facilitators, based on the Transcultural Model, would work as a team. The organization of the team could be similar to that of Doctors without Borders. It would be made up of carefully selected Indigenous and non-Indigenous persons who are role models, perhaps already working in the human services field. Commitment to their own personal healing journey would be a basic requirement.

▶ The curriculum would be based on experiential learning, team members participating as a group in each segment of the model. After each session, they would analyze the group's interactions: what went well, what didn't, what could have been done differently? Their training would also acquaint them with the basic knowledge, skills and attitudes for working in a community, knowing when to make appropriate referrals to other community agencies.

▶ Additional training modules could be developed that would be offered in conjunction with the Transcultural Healing Model, especially ones dealing with human energy fields, nutrition and body care.

▶ A program for *Community Transition Consultants* could be developed. Its purpose would be to train community specialists who could assist communities in translating their Community Vision into a blueprint for action and implementation. They would need to be familiar with governmental and non-governmental resources, seeking out opportunities to form partnerships between Indigenous and non-Indigenous segments of society.

▶ Indigenous Elders could be available for advice, teaching, counselling, and inspiring the trainees, as well as providing advice on the development of the Community Healing Institute.

▶ Transcultural communications weekends could be offered, made up of a mix of Indigenous and non-Indigenous persons. The purpose would be to conduct experiential exercises that would facilitate seeing one's self in the other. This can be done through music, art, relaxation and visualizations and quiet times in togetherness.

In summary, *the fundamental principles and practices of healing are transcultural.* The concepts and exercises that have been outlined here can be applied to any group or community that wants to undergo a healing process. Canada is now in a transition period, trying to redefine the relationship between the Indigenous and non-Indigenous segments of society. Much needs to be done; however, attitude change cannot be legislated, nor do people change their negative stereotypes easily. It is only through a nonjudgmental experience of the *Other* that hearts can change and eyes be opened to our shared humanness.

"In a circle, the end is a new beginning."

POSTSCRIPT

My book, *Community Healing: A Transcultural Model,* ended with the words, "In a circle, the end is a new beginning." Perhaps those words were predictive. Now that the book is being readied for publishing, I feel the need to add a postscript to the model outlined in these pages.

In the beginning of my book, community is described as being a collection of individuals plus "something more"— an extensive web of relationships and ways of being that evolved over the centuries. It was this web that was eroded by a "foreign" intrusion, as the European culture exerted dominance over individuals and communities, initiating a process of dis-integration and dis-ease. Community healing, starting with its individual members, is the main focus of this book.

And yet, there is another, larger web, one that has also been, and still is, in the process of dis-integration and dis-ease. This web comprises the totality of the overall environment within which individuals and communities exist, a massive ecosystem.

An ecosystem is defined as being "a biological community of interacting organisms and their physical environment." It is a complex, inter-connected and dynamic web of relationships: individuals within their communities, communities with each other, all existing within their natural, physical environment.

Just as "no man is an island," no community exists in isolation of this larger reality, its ecosystem. In fact, the larger reality inter-penetrates the community and its individuals at all levels. In this way, the well-being of the individual, the community and the environment are intrinsically interlinked with each other. Increasing the quality of the well-being of one aspect of this ecosystem increases the well-being of all the other components as well. Degrading the quality of one aspect is to degrade, or destroy, the well-being of the other levels.

There is an emerging sense that the health and well-being of the world ecosystem is no longer "well," that, without action, it will continue to collapse to the point where life for many will no longer be sustainable. This has already occurred for many Indigenous communities. How can Humpty Dumpty be put back together again?

For healing to take place, Indigenous and non-Indigenous people must first become *aware* that we are all a part of a massive, endangered, ecosystem--that what we think and how we act in our every-day lives affects the whole. The second necessary requirement is for all of us to *assume responsibility* for ourselves and our shared ecosystem--and be willing to change our behaviours. The third necessary requirement is *to act*.

The Truth and Reconciliation Commission has called upon all levels of government, from the federal to the municipal, to develop a national action plan that will reconcile government policies with responsible action, especially in relation to how *traditional values* relate to *guardianship, stewardship and sustainability* of the land—*our* land.

In the Anishinabek News, 12/20/15, Elder Mary Deleary, is quoted:

> *The responsibilities that our ancestors carried ... are still being carried .... Even through all of the struggles, even through all of what has been disrupted, we can still hear the voices of the land. The land is made up of the dust of our ancestors' bones. And so, to reconcile with this land and everything that has happened, there is much work to be done. (edited)*

Where to start? This book provides a transcultural model which, if implemented, will initiate a process of change and healing at the micro-level, that of the individual and the community.

Change at the macro level is much more complicated as the voices of those in power are often at odds with the "voices of the land." However, if we as a nation wake up and begin to realize that our very survival is embedded in the well-being and preservation of our ecosystem, then a blueprint for all decision-making at whatever level should emerge, based on values intrinsic to survival and sustainability.

Chief Dan George was wise when he advised us to:

Keep a few embers
From the fire
That used to burn in your village,
Someday go back
So all can gather again
And rekindle a new flame,
For a new life in a changed world.

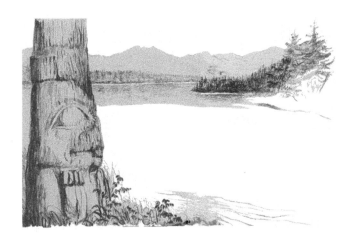

JUGGEJTIONJ FOR BACK-GROUND JTUDY

Allender, Don. *The Wounded Heart.* Colorado Springs: Navpress, 1990.

Attenborough, Richard. "There is a light," www.goodreads.com, no date.

Bellegarde, Chief Perry, quoted in "National Strategy on Suicide Needed," *The Okanagan,* March 12, 2016, p. A 6.

Berne, Eric, M.D. *Games People Play.* New York: Ballentine Books, 1964.

Chung, Stan, "Discrimination Stops When Everyone Becomes White," *The Daily Courier,* January 15, 2017, p. A 8.

Dunham, Arthur. *The New Community Organization.* New York: Thomas Y. Crowell Company, 1970.

Eastcott, Michal. *"I, the Story of the Self."* Wheaton: Theosophical Publishing, 1980.

Erasmus, Peter and Geneva Ensign. *Practical Framework for Community Liaison Work.* Brandon, Manitoba: J.P. Publishing, 1991.

Gibran, Kahlil. *The Prophet.* New York: Alfred A. Knopf, 1980.

Hamachek, D.E. *Encounters with the Self* (2nd Ed.). New York: Holt, Rinehart and Winston, 1978.

Heckbert, Doug. "The Indigenous Experience: Is It Important To Know About This?" *Justice Actualites Report*, Volume 28, No. 2, pp. 18-27.

Jacobi, Jolande. *The Psychology of C. G. Jung.* New Haven: Yale University Press, 1973.

Jung, Carl. *Memories, Dreams and Reflections.* New York: Vintage, 1989.

Jung, Carl. *The Undiscovered Self.* New York: New American Library, 1958.

Kermayer, Dr. Laurence, quoted in "Attawapiskat Crisis: Rash of Suicide Attempts Could be a Chain Reaction," *The Daily Courier,* April 14, 2016, p. A 4.

Lifton, R. J. *The Life of the Self: Toward a New Psychology.* New York: Basic Books, Inc., 1983.

Mails, Thomas E. *Fools Crow.* Lincoln: University of Nebraska Press, 1979.

Mails, Thomas E. *Fools Crow: Wisdom and Power.* San Francisco: Council Oaks Books, 1991.

Metcalfe-Chenail, Danielle, ed. *In This Together: Fifteen Stories of Truth & Reconciliation.* Victoria: Brindle & Glass Publishing, 2016.

Nisbet, Robert A. *The Quest for Community.* London: Oxford University Press, 1953.

Olien, Glenn. "The 33 Community Supports: Unified Community Transition Theory," *Employment Self-Assessment Tool*, British Columbia, 1996.

Osborne, Cecil. *Understanding Your Past: Key to Your Future.* Nashville: Abingdon Press, 1980.

Peck, Scott. *A World Waiting to Be Born.* New York: Bantam Books, 1993.

Rogers, Carl. *On Personal Power.* Delicorte Press, 1977.

Selye, Hans, M.D. *Stress without Distress.* Scarborough: The New American Library of Canada, Ltd., 1975.

Stonechild, Blair. Regina: University of Regina Press, 2016.

"Truth and Reconciliation Commission Canada: Calls to Action." Truth and Reconciliation Commission of Canada, Public Domain, Winnipeg, 2015.

SUGGESTED BOOKS TO DISPLAY DURING HEALING CIRCLES

Benson, H. *The Relaxation Response.* New York: William Morrow and Company, 1975.

Brachet, Michelle. *Little Book of Reflexology.* U.K.: Demand Media, 2013.

Brown, Joseph, Ed. *The Sacred Pipe.* New York: Penguin Books, 1977.

Brown, Les. *Live Your Dreams.* New York: Harper Collins, 1992.

Bryne, Hugh. *The Here and Now Habit.* Oakland, California: New Harbinger, 1997.

Chief Dan George. *My Heart Soars*. Toronto: Hancock House Publishers, Ltd., 1974.

Chief Dan George. *My Spirit Soars*. Toronto: Hancock House Publishers, Ltd., 1982.

Gordon, Richard. *Your Healing Hands*. Santa Cruz: Unity Press, 1978.

Kinew, Wab. *The Reason You Walk*. New York: Viking Press, 2015.

Lane, Phil, Jr., Judie & Michael Bopp, Lee Brown & Elders. *The Sacred Tree*. Twin Lakes, Wisconsin: Lotus Press, 2012.

Parke, Simon. *One Minute Mindfulness*. UK: Hay House, 2013.

Solomon, Arthur. *Songs for the People: Teachings on the Natural Way*. Toronto: New Canada Publications, 1992.

Wagamese, Richard. *Embers: One Ojibway's Meditations*. Madeira Park, BC: Douglas and McIntyre, 2016.

SUGGESTIONS FOR HEALING CIRCLE MUSIC

The records and tapes listed below are ones, among others, that I have used repeatedly in workshops for relaxation exercises as well as for background music. Music in 4/4 time slows the heart rate.

▶ Zamfir: *The Lonely Shepherd*. Polydor.

▶ *Old Agency Singers of the Blood Reserve*. Indian House.

▶ Canyon Records. Northern Cree Singers: Drumming

▶ Red Bull Singers: *Mother Earth*

▶ Hagood Hardy: *The Homecoming*. Attic.

▶ Johann Sebastian Bach: *Harpsichord Concertos, Vol. 3*. Angel.

▶ Andres Segovia: *The Intimate Guitar*. R.C.A.

▶ Danny Wright: *Autumn Dreams*.

▶ John St. John: *Loon Lake*.

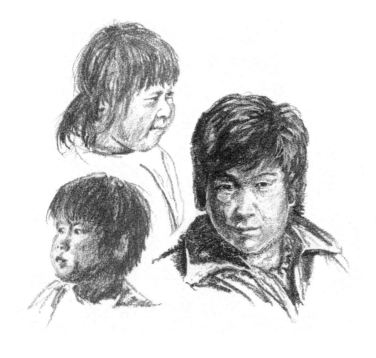

APPENDICES

APPENDIX 1

EXERCISES AND TECHNIQUES*

IN GENERAL

▶ Encourage individuals to express their feelings directly, rather than *talking about* their feelings. This can be done by asking them to talk aloud to whoever hurt them, using present tense and the word "I," as in, "I am angry…" "I am hurt." A puppet, a pillow, a chair can be used as a stand-in for whomever they are talking to.

▶ When working with a dream, guided visualization or a picture, have them become each part of it and see what awarenesses emerge. For example, "I am a mountain. I am tall, strong, eternal. I can't be worn down."

▶ Ask open-ended questions, like:

> ❯ *You are angry because…*

> ❯ *What are you feeling right now?*

> ❯ *What colour is your feeling?*

> ❯ *What shape is your feeling?*

> ❯ *How old is this feeling?*

> ➤ *You said that...*

> ➤ *Go beneath the feeling. What's there?*

▶ Draw awareness to their body language, a manifestation of their feeling, for example, clenched fists or teeth, closed eyes, hand over mouth. Make suggestions like:

> ➤ *Imagine putting your feelings into your arm; your fist: If it could talk, what would it say?*

> ➤ *Put your hand where the feeling is. Let the feeling be there. It's okay to feel... Allow the feeling to happen.*

> ➤ *It's okay to talk now. You don't have to be silent any more.*

> ➤ *Say that again, louder ... louder ... louder.*

▶ Allow whatever is happening to happen; don't interrupt unless you sense that the person cannot handle the depth of emotion. If so, gently suggest some type of closure "for now." They can wrap up in a blanket, curl up in a chair, whatever seems appropriate in the moment for comfort.

▶ Following a unit of work, it is helpful to ensure the client "comes back" to the "now." Specific questions will bring the individual back to thinking, rather than feeling. For example, *When you get back home, what specifically will you do?*

▶ Reinforce the importance of "I" statements. I am ... I will ... I won't. Using "I" statements promotes self-responsibility and brings the person to the present, not the maybes of the future.

▶ Work with symbolic meaning of words rather than literal meanings. Not everyone is ready to work with symbolism, but the facilitator should always try. Metaphoric meaning is more powerful than literal meaning and brings latent material from the unconscious to the conscious.

TECHNIQUES FOR MOVING BLOCKED ENERGY

▶ Deep breathing

▶ Fantasy trip through body

▶ Stress position; increase the tension in what already feels tight

▶ Neck tension release

▶ Be a rag doll

▶ Energy in hands; play with "ball of energy;" feel the magnetic pull

▶ Hitting a pillow or couch, encouraging sounds

▶ Foot, back, neck massage

▶ Bring their awareness to physical manifestations of feeling, such as clenched fists, closed eyes

▶ Have them imagine putting feelings into fist, arm, etc. Have fist "talk;" give it a motion.

ADDITIONAL EXERCISES

All experiential exercises include an activity, chosen to bring a specific awareness, followed by the processing of the personal feelings and awarenesses that were catalyzed by that activity—individually and collectively as a group. Some of these are extremely helpful if members are having trouble relaxing and feeling comfortable as a group.

TRUST WALK

In twos. One partner is blindfolded. Instructions: *You are to take your partner on a walk without talking. You may hold their arm, but you cannot talk. You are to prove that you are trustworthy and your partner's job is to learn to trust. Both of you should stay aware of feelings. At the end of the walk, change positions, still without talking. When you are finished, share with each other what you experienced.*

Report back as a team what happened and how you felt. How does it feel to trust another person?

TREE FANTASY

Instructions: *Stand up straight, both feet solidly on the ground/floor. You are a tree. Feel your branches; feel the breeze blowing through your leaves. What kind of tree are you? Become aware of your roots. How deep do they go? Be aware of your taproot, the main one that feeds you. Let your awareness follow it deep into the ground. Feel your connection with Mother Earth and Mother Sky.*

MEET SELF OF THE FUTURE

Choose a time in the future. What do you look like? What are you wearing? What are you doing? How do you feel? What have you accomplished?

ON BEING ALONE

What is it like to be alone? Do you always have to be around people, on your phone or busy with being busy? Choose somewhere in the room that is separate from the others. Sit down on the floor. Take a deep breath, close your eyes, and "feel" your aloneness. Pretend that there is no one around for miles. Be aware of your feelings and your body language.

Group go-round: *What did you experience? Is there a difference between aloneness and being lonely?*

IF I HAD MY LIFE TO LIVE OVER

Read poem to the group.

If I had my life to live over,
I'd dare to make more mistakes next time.
I'd relax,
I would limber up.
I would be sillier than I have been on this trip.
I would take fewer things seriously.
I would take more chances.
I would climb more mountains and swim more rivers.
I would eat more ice cream and less beans.
I would perhaps have more actual troubles,
But I would have fewer imaginary ones.
You see, I am one of those people
Who live sensibly and sanely hour after hour,

Day after day.
Oh, I've had my moments
And if I had it to do over again,
I'd have more of them.
In fact, I would try to have nothing but moments,
Just moments, one after another,
Instead of living so many years ahead of each day.
I've been one of those persons who
Never goes anywhere without a thermometer,
A hot water bottle, a raincoat and a
Parachute.
If I had to do it again, I would travel
Lighter than I have.
If I had my life to life over,
I would start barefoot earlier in the spring
And stay that way later in the fall.
I would go to more dances;
I would ride more merry-go-rounds,
I would pick more daisies.

–Nadine Stair, an 85-year-old woman from Kentucky

Make a list of what you would do over if you could. Share your list with your small group.

YOU ARE RESPONSIBLE FOR YOUR SURVIVAL

Jot down the things that you do to take care of each of your needs:

▶ *Your body?*

▶ *Your mind?*

▶ *Your feelings?*

▶ *Your spirit?*

Go back to put a + sign by the things you do that are life-giving for yourself. Put a – sign by those things that are not good for you. Reflect on what things you should/could do to take better care of yourself. What will you do differently?

DRAWING OF SELF

▶ *Choose a partner with whom you are comfortable. One person lies down on a large sheet of butcher paper. The partner draws around the body, both persons being aware of their feelings. Switch positions and outline the other person's body.*

▶ *Cut yourself out; again, be aware at all times of what you are feeling. What made you uncomfortable? Why? What made you comfortable, happy?*

▶ *Draw your physical scars; what unresolved emotions are involved in the scar?*

▶ *In your heart area, draw a symbol that stands for you at your most alive, vibrant self (Spirit). Use bright colours. Gold, silver and white felt-tips can be used as well.*

▶ *Using masking tape, attach your image to the wall. Look at yourself from a distance. What do you see? Would you want this person as a best friend?*

▶ *Introduce yourself to the group.*

▶ During this exercise, the facilitator should be aware of how each person is doing. Walk around, being encouraging and aware of what's happening. Who is too careful, careless, emotional? In one workshop, a person crumpled up the picture and threw it under a chair. One action spoke a thousand words.

WHAT MOTIVATES YOUR LIFE?

Have the group lie down on the floor on blankets. Talk about life as being breath, motion, and action. Have them hold their breath as long as they can and then ask the questions:

▶ *What beckons you?*

▶ *What entices you to get up?*

▶ *Why do you get up in the morning?*

▶ *What things make you feel alive?*

▶ *What things make you feel dead, slow, heavy?*

EXPERIENCING STRESS

▶ *Squat on your toes with your back against the wall. Hold position as long as possible. What do you become aware of in your body, your mind, your feelings? When else do you feel like this?*

MY CO-WORKER AND MY COLLEAGUE— "ME"

▶ *In your journal, jot down all the words that describe a person whom you do not like to work with. Why? What bothers you?*

▶ *Now jot down all the words that describe a person who you would like to work with. What is it that you like?*

▶ *Now, claim everyone of those words, putting "I am..." in front. Do any of these describe you?*

DEATH AS AN ADVISOR

▶ *Write your full name—all the names you have ever used. What feelings do you have about your names?*

▶ *Draw your lifeline, as illustrated below.*

▶ *Date of Birth _____ X _____ Death*

▶ *Make an "x" on the lifeline, marking when you think/feel you will die. How?*

▶ *What do you think happens after death?*

WHAT WILL PEOPLE SAY AT YOUR FUNERAL?

▶ *Imagine your own funeral. What are people saying? What would you like them to say? What would you say to them if you could?*

▶ *If you had _____ time to live, what would you do differently?*

▶ *Are you aware of anything that you could/should do now so you will not have any regrets when your time does come?*

ENERGIZER OR ICEBREAKER: "HOW DO YOU LIKE YOUR NEIGHBOUR?"

▶ Circle of chairs. *Who will volunteer to be It? It does not have a chair. It chooses someone and stands before that person, asking, "How do you like your neighbours?"*

▶ *The person chosen gives the names of the persons on each side of them, saying, "I like my neighbours fine; I like Amanda and I like Carl, but I do not like people with glasses or black shoes or... .*

▶ *Everyone with ____ must get up and find another chair, but not a chair on either side of their original seat.*

▶ *The one who does not find a chair is now It.*

▶ *However, if It says, "No, I do not like my neighbors," everyone must find new seats.*

▶ Ten minutes of this game gets people energized, laughing and ready to go again!

* Created or Collected by Geneva Ensign, 2017

APPENDIX 2

AN EFFECTIVE GROUP

► Has a clear understanding of its purposes and goals

► Has members who trust each other; members feel free to share ideas, feelings and opinions

► Is one where all members have feelings of belonging (community)

► Has agreed-upon ways of doing things, including rituals and ceremonies

► Has good discussions, where ideas are clarified by asking open-ended questions

► Makes decisions while considering all viewpoints, reaching agreement and commitment

► Achieves a balance between getting the job done and meeting the emotional needs of its members

► Shares leadership

► Is okay with differences of opinion; members can agree to disagree

► Can talk about team problems, focusing on the issue, not attacking the person

► Works from a wholistic framework: body, mind, feelings and spirit

► Has fun; its members enjoy being together

Adapted from Lippitt and Whitefield

APPENDIX 3

BEHAVIOURS RESULTING FROM SELF-LOVE OR SELF-HATE

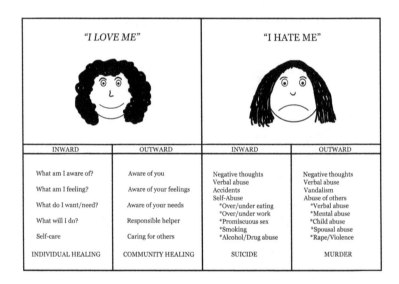

"I LOVE ME"		"I HATE ME"	
INWARD	OUTWARD	INWARD	OUTWARD
What am I aware of?	Aware of you	Negative thoughts	Negative thoughts
What am I feeling?	Aware of your feelings	Verbal abuse	Verbal abuse
What do I want/need?	Aware of your needs	Accidents	Vandalism
What will I do?	Responsible helper	Self-Abuse	Abuse of others
Self-care	Caring for others	*Over/under eating	*Verbal abuse
		*Over/under work	*Mental abuse
		*Promiscuous sex	*Child abuse
		*Smoking	*Spousal abuse
		*Alcohol/Drug abuse	*Rape/Violence
INDIVIDUAL HEALING	COMMUNITY HEALING	SUICIDE	MURDER

APPENDIX 4

	Behaviours That Help	Behaviours That Hinder
Verbal		
Non-Verbal		

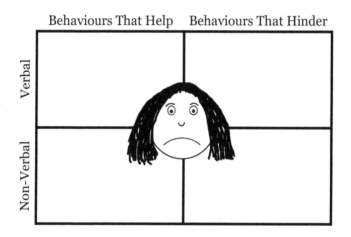

APPENDIX 5

COMMUNITY PLANNING PRINCIPLES

PRINCIPLES:

▶ Every person in a community is valuable and *has inherent worth and dignity.*

▶ *Self-determination* is a basic right and responsibility of individuals and groups, meaning the ability to make decisions individually and with others for the good of the group.

▶ Within each person are *the desire and ability*, to learn, grow and develop.

▶ Growth implies *positive development* in all aspects of one's self: Body, Mind, Feelings, and Spirit.

▶ Each individual has a unique contribution to make to the *life* of a community.

▶ Community change *happens* as individuals within it grow and change.

THEREFORE, COMMUNITY PLANNING WILL:

▶ Be concerned with the overall well-being of all community members

▶ Be concerned with facilitating growth by deliberate, conscious action and planning

▶ Integrate and use knowledge and expertise from all disciplines

▶ Work with community people in various combinations: individuals, one-to-one, small groups, inter-group and the community as a whole

▶ Be based in self-help and self-responsibility

▶ Be based in participation, involvement and cooperative action

▶ Work with self and/or community-identified issues, not pre-determined agendas

▶ Use conscious decision-making or general agreement, not majority win

▶ Emphasize process (people participation and cooperation) over a predetermined result

▶ Be long-term, not a crash program

Adapted from Dunham, 1970, pp. 172-173.

APPENDIX 6

EVALUATION
COMMUNITY HEALING
CIRCLE

1. Given the goals for the workshop, how would you rate your experience?

Poor	Fair	Good	Very Good	Excellent

2. What sessions were most helpful to you?

Poor	Fair	Good	Very Good	Excellent

3. What would you like to have been different?

Poor	Fair	Good	Very Good	Excellent

4. How did you personally benefit from these sessions?

Poor	Fair	Good	Very Good	Excellent

5. What words come to mind when you think of the workshop?

Poor	Fair	Good	Very Good	Excellent

Other comments?

Name of Workshop: _____

Facilitator: _____

Date: _____

APPENDIX 7

HOW CAN I TELL YOU WHAT YOU MAY NOT WANT TO HEAR?

W E ARE NOT alone in this world; we are born into families and into communities. We need each other to survive; yet, we usually are never taught how to talk to the people in our lives.

Most of us have trouble trying to tell someone something that person might not want to hear. Below are some helpful hints for giving "feedback" to another person:

► Use the word "I" as in: "I feel..."; "I think..."; "I would like..."; "I don't like..."; "I don't want...". By using the word "I," you are taking responsibility for yourself. You are not making demands. That leaves the other person free to say what they feel and want. Then you can find a solution based on real feelings and desires; both of you can "win."

► Describe the other person's behaviour; don't judge or evaluate it.

► Share your own feelings about what is happening. Ask the other person to share their feelings.

► Be as specific as possible, rather than general.

▶ Find a good time to talk with someone when it is about them. Wait until they are ready to "hear" you.

▶ Check your own reason for giving feedback. If in doubt about your own motivation, wait!

▶ Don't forget! You can tell someone something that you *do* like. When was the last time you told someone they looked great? Or that you appreciated the work they are doing? Or that the meal was wonderful? Or that their smile gave you a new start on the day?

▶ Positive feedback can be nonverbal as well—a smile, a pat, a hug...

▶ Remember the old saying, "You can catch more flies with honey than with vinegar."

APPENDIX 8

IMPACT OF PERSONAL AWARENESS SESSIONS

Native Counselling Services of Alberta
Doug Heckbert

I WORKED WITH NATIVE Counselling Services of Alberta in Edmonton from 1976 to 1983 as a staff trainer, training coordinator and program director. My principal focus was on assessing and meeting the training needs of all staff.

Initially, I concentrated on the field staff (court workers and prison liaison workers), then the office staff (secretaries, receptionists and bookkeepers) and then administrative staff (supervisors and program directors).

What I noticed initially about the field staff is what terrific people they were. This confirmed my earlier experiences with many Aboriginal people. They were hard-working, dedicated to NCSA, well respected in their communities and focused on doing a good job for their clients. I noticed, however, that many tended to make self-deprecating comments, leading me to think might be an issue of a lack of self-confidence. The staff tended to be negative about themselves. This did not make much sense to me, given the skills and knowledge I saw these folks demonstrate. I wondered about the possibility that I was seeing something that might be a cultural trait, or was it more of a personal feature? Eventually, I decided it was far more personal than cultural, and I turned my attention to how I could approach the matter from a training perspective.

Prior to working at NCSA, I worked for Alberta Corrections and the National Parole Service. I knew quite a few criminal justice officials that would be working with the court workers and prison liaison staff. In discussing training issues with these officials and listening to the staff talk about what they thought would help them in their work, one theme emerged other than issues related to law, policy and programs. That theme was personal development. As I talked more about this topic with staff and officials and read some of the training literature, it started to become clear that finding ways to help staff increase their knowledge of their values, strengths, and capabilities would translate into them becoming more self-confident, more assertive and thus more effective in their work.

The late 1970s and early 1980s were turbulent times for Canadians and Aboriginal people. I heard a lot of put-downs of Native people, assertions as to their inability to work and comments about their racial inferiority. The constitutional discussions and the notion of Aboriginal self-government brought new focus and attention to Aboriginal issues. It was during this time that I learned some details about residential schools from Aboriginal staff that had attended or knew others that had. I was appalled by some of the details I heard. As I spent more time with the staff, I began to realize the extent to which Aboriginal people had been held apart and marginalized from mainstream society for many generations. I concluded it was no wonder that many Aboriginal people internalized negative views of themselves, their families and their communities. I was comfortable that I could see why many staff seemed to hold negative personal attitudes.

The question then became: what can I do about this? One possible answer emerged, and that would be to promote training sessions that focused on personal awareness and personal development, where participants would unlearn some of the "negative stuff" they had internalized and replace those negative attitudes with positive ones.

I began searching for resources that I could work with. One such resource was Grant MacEwan Community College in Edmonton. The college was founded in 1971 to focus on the educational needs of communities and community groups by offering college-level programs that focused on career development. Initial educational offerings included one-year certificate and two-year diploma programs. The various programs offered credit and non-credit courses on-site and by outreach courses contracted to community-based educational authorities and agencies. I discovered that the Social Work program offered personal development courses taught by qualified instructors and that the non-credit courses could be tailored to the needs of the participants.

Over the years, several instructors from MacEwan ran personal awareness for NCSA. I took part in many of these sessions and ensured that the other training staff took part as well. One particular instructor stood out, in my mind, and that was Geneva Ensign. I had met Geneva several years before at the University of Alberta, when she was studying for a master's degree in community development and I was working on a master's in sociology (corrections).

I deliberately chose the wording "Personal Awareness" as the title for the sessions rather than "Personal Development." To my way of thinking, staff would respond more positively to the idea of becoming aware of themselves rather than developing themselves, the latter term could be taken negatively, i.e., *What is wrong with me?"*

Geneva had a wonderful way of relating with the NCSA staff. Although she was Caucasian, she had a very good understanding of the Aboriginal experience in Canada, including the negative impact on the emotional wellbeing of many Aboriginal people. She was supportive, encouraging, and upbeat, and she gently pushed the staff to "be themselves" and to let others see what terrific people they were. All the structured activities were carefully explained, respectfully carried out and thoroughly debriefed under Geneva's guidance. In every session, there were tears, laughter, and "aha!" moments when someone realized what insight they gained as to their personal awareness and strengths.

As a result of attending a five-day personal awareness session, most staff came away:

► showing more confidence in themselves as individuals and as Aboriginal persons

► with increased understanding and acceptance of the other participants

► with increased assertiveness both personally and in terms of their work with NCSA

► expressing a more positive outlook on the organization's goals, philosophy, mission and programs

Not everyone responded so positively. A few staff expressed neutral feelings in their assessment of the sessions ("Yeah, it was okay, but I could have accomplished more by staying at home and going to work."). A small number of staff, I believe, were really challenged by what they learned about themselves, and they did not like what they saw. "That was a waste of time—I won't be doing that again."

On a personal level, I thoroughly enjoyed the sessions with Geneva. I felt closer to the staff and I believed they came to know me better. One comment still comes to mind many years later—a statement from Nora, a Cree woman from northern Alberta, about me, a White guy: "Doug, you are a good Indian!" These words made my day, and I believe they speak volumes as to how far both Nora and I came in that few days together under Geneva's guidance. In my view, we came more aware of ourselves and of each other, and in doing so, we developed as better persons who made better contributions to our organization.

APPENDIX 9

SUPPLIES NEEDED FOR HEALING CIRCLES	CHAPTERS				
	8	9	10	11	12
Balls of strong string, red, green, yellow			x		
Blanket for each person	x	x			
Books: Inspirational, Indigenous, Relaxation	x	x	x	x	x
Books: Body care, Massage	x	x	x	x	x
Box felt tip pens for each person, basic colours	x	x	x	x	x
Box tissue	x	x	x	x	x
Candle, matches, tray	x	x	x	x	x
Circles, white paper, 8" diameter			x		
Coffee/tea/water/juices/goodies	x		x	x	x
Construction paper, all colours			x		
Duo tangs (journals), lined, unlined paper	x	x	x	x	x
Evaluation Forms	x	x	x	x	x
Flip chart & flip chart paper	x	x	x	x	x
Gifts for each person, small, symbolic	x	x	x	x	x
Gold, silver, white liner pens	x	x	x	x	x
Legal size paper, white	x	x	x	x	x
Masking tape & glue stick	x	x	x	x	x
Music player	x	x	x	x	x
Music, variety, 4x4 beat - drumming, flute, classical	x	x	x	x	x
Music, variety, upbeat music for break time	x	x	x	x	x
Name tags	x	x	x	x	x
Pens or pencils	x	x	x	x	x
Pillow for each person, floor sitting	x	x	x	x	x
Scissors	x	x	x	x	x
Sign-In sheet, with names, phone #, e-mail	x	x	x	x	x
HANDOUTS:					
An Effective Group				x	
Behaviours Resulting from Self-Hate or Self-Love		x			
Behaviours That Help or Hinder Working Together				x	
Community Planning Principles					x
I Love Me/I Hate Me		x			
T.A. Model with 2 circles, 4 for each person			x		
To Know How You Are Acting, Listen to Your Words			x		

APPENDIX 10

TO KNOW HOW YOU'RE ACTING,
LISTEN TO YOUR WORDS

ACTING LIKE A PARENT - THE AUTHORITY FIGURE
(INSTRUCTING, DECIDING, TELLING, TAKING CARE OF)

YOU SHOULD   YOU OUGHT   YOU MUST   YOU HAVE TO
LET ME TELL YOU   LISTEN TO ME!   I'M THE BOSS
DO WHAT I SAY   I KNOW BEST   DON'T DO THAT
WHEN WILL YOU GROW UP?   LET ME DO IT: YOU DON'T KNOW HOW
IF YOU DON'T DO WHAT I SAY, THEN I WILL...   WE WILL DO IT THIS WAY
DON'T DO WHAT I DO; DO WHAT I SAY!   I'M RIGHT! YOU'RE WRONG!
I'LL TAKE CARE OF IT/YOU   DO IT THE RIGHT WAY - MY WAY!

ACTING LIKE A CHILD - THE PLEASER
(DEPENDENT, CLINGING, WHINING, SUBSERVIENT, HELPLESS)

SO SORRY   PLEASE DO IT FOR ME   I'M MISUNDERSTOOD
YES, YES   I WON'T EVER DO IT AGAIN   I'M LONELY   TAKE CARE OF ME
I CAN'T DO IT   LET ME MAKE YOU HAPPY   I'LL BE QUIET
I'LL HELP YOU - IF YOU'LL LOVE ME   LOOK AT ME   SEE ME   I CAN'T
I'LL FIX IT, DON'T WORRY   I CAN'T   I'LL PAY FOR IT   DON'T BE ANGRY
LOVE ME   IS IT O.K.?   I'M UGLY   I'M NO GOOD   DID I DO IT RIGHT?

ACTING LIKE A CHILD - THE REBEL
(EXTREMELY INDEPENDENT, RAGING, BLAMING, ACCUSING,
BULLYING, SNEAKY, MANIPULATING)

YOU MADE ME DO IT   I WON'T   YOU CAN'T MAKE ME DO IT! NO!
YOU'RE UGLY   YOU'RE NO GOOD   I'LL DO IT WHEN I FEEL LIKE IT
YOU'RE NOT MY BOSS   I'M TOO BUSY   "BUG OFF!"   I HATE YOU
MY WAY OR THE HIGHWAY   IT'S YOUR FAULT   I WANT IT RIGHT NOW!

ACTING LIKE AN ADULT - THE SELF-RESPONSIBLE GROWN-UP
(INTER-DEPENDENT, CARES FOR SELF AND OTHERS)

I WILL   I CHOOSE NOT TO   I WILL LISTEN TO YOU
I WON'T JUDGE YOU   WHAT DO YOU NEED/WANT?
I WON'T DO IT FOR YOU, BUT I WILL SHOW YOU HOW

Geneva Ensign, 2017

APPENDIX 11

TRANSCULTURAL COMMUNITY HEALING PROCESS: PROGRESS REPORT

On a scale of 1 to 5, rate your community planning process in terms of the following criteria.
1 Indicates very little has been done; 5 would mean that aspect has been very well covered.

1. REQUEST FOR A HEALING PROCESS CAME FROM THE COMMUNITY

   1 2 3 4 5

2. TOP-LEVEL DECISION MAKERS ARE ON BOARD WITH IDEA

   1 2 3 4 5

3. AN OVERALL INDIVIDUAL & COMMUNITY HEALING PLAN HAS BEEN DEVELOPED

   1 2 3 4 5

4. HEALING PLAN BASED ON TRANSCULTURAL VALUES

   1 2 3 4 5

5. EMPHASIS ON COMMUNITY HEALING PERMEATES ALL DECISIONS & PROGRAMMING

   1 2 3 4 5

6. AVAILABLE TO ALL COMMUNITY MEMBERS WHO CHOOSE TO ATTEND

   1 2 3 4 5

7. BASED ON INDIVIDUAL CHOICE AND COOPERATIVE ACTION

   1 2 3 4 5

8. WORKS WITH THE POSITIVE, PROMOTING STRENGTHS

   1 2 3 4 5

9. USES COMMUNITY RESOURCES AS MUCH AS POSSIBLE

   1 2 3 4 5

10. TRAINING CORE GROUP OF FACILITATORS, WITH ON-GOING TRAINING

    1 2 3 4 5

11. BRINGS PEOPLE TOGETHER IN VARIOUS COMBINATIONS

    1 2 3 4 5

12. FACILITATES COOPERATION & TEAMWORK AMONG ALL DEPARTMENTS

    1 2 3 4 5

13. SEEN AS LONG TERM; TIME FRAME BASED ON ACTUAL NEED, NOT PRE-DETERMINED

    1 2 3 4 5

14. ON-GOING EVALUATION PROCESS THAT GUIDES & INFORMS NEXT STEPS

    1 2 3 4 5

15. FUNDING ADEQUATE, FLEXIBLE, ADAPTABLE TO CHANGING NEEDS

    1 2 3 4 5

Adapted from Dunham, 1970

APPENDIX 12

"The Red Deer Connection" was given to me by the artist, Geraldine Crop Eared Wolf, following a 1980s workshop in Alberta. She said that it depicted the rainbow of love that had woven all the participants together in the circle. This was particularly significant because it was a meeting between traditional enemies, the Bloods and the Crees, who were now in training to be social workers.

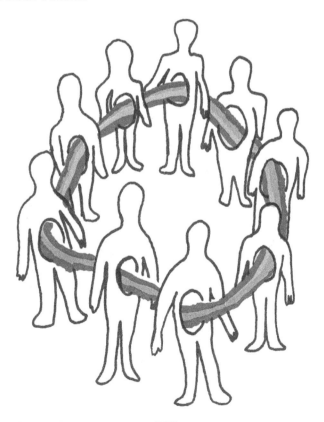

INDEX

A

B

C

P

Q

R

S

Y

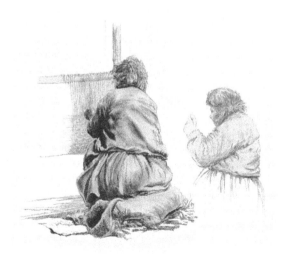

other Indigenous culture titles from **HANCOCK HOUSE PUBLISHERS**

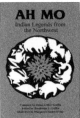 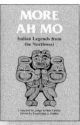 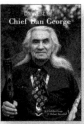 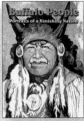 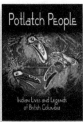

Ah Mo
Tren Griffin
978-0-88839-244-2
5½ x 8½, sc, 64 pp
$7.95

More Ah Mo
Tren Griffin
978-0-88839-303-6
5½ x 8½, sc, 64 pp
$7.95

The Best of Chief Dan George
978-0-88839-544-3
5½ x 8½, sc, 216 pp
$12.95

Buffalo People
Mildred Valley Thornton
978-0-88839-479-8
5½ x 8½, sc, 208 pp
$24.95

Potlatch People
Mildred Valley Thornton
978-0-88839-491-0
5½ x 8½, sc, 320pp
$24.95

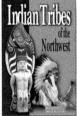 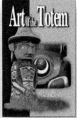 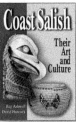 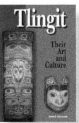 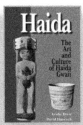

Indian Tribes
Reg Ashwell
David Hancock
978-0-88839-619-8
full color, 5½ x 8½, sc, 96 pp
$11.95

Art of the Totem
Marius Barbeau
David Hancock
978-0-88839-618-1
full color, 5½ x 8½, sc, 64 pp
$9.95

Coast Salish
Reg Ashwell
David Hancock
978-0-88839-620-4
full color, 5½ x 8½, sc, 96 pp
$11.95

Tlingit
David Hancock
978-0-88839-530-2
5½ x 8½, sc, 96 pp
$12.95

Haida
Leslie Drew,
David Hancock
978-0-88839-621-X
full color 5½ x 8½, sc, 96 pp
$12.95

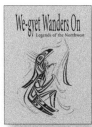 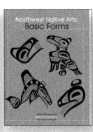 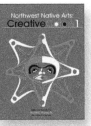 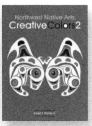

We-gyet Wanders On
Kitanmax School of Northwest Coast Art
978-0-88839-636-5
8½ x 11, sc, 72 pp
$14.95

Basic Forms
Robert E. Stanley Sr.
978-0-88839-506-1
8½ x 11, sc, 64 pp
$11.95

Creative Colors 1
Robert E. Stanley Sr.
978-0-88839-532-0
8½ x 11, sc, 32 pp
$6.95

Creative Colors 2
Robert E. Stanley Sr.
978-0-88839-533-7
8½ x 11, sc, 24 pp
$5.95

Hancock House Publishers
19313 0 Ave, Surrey, BC V3Z 9R9
www.hancockhouse.com
sales@hancockhouse.com
1-800-938-1114

CPSIA information can be obtained
at www.ICGtesting.com
Printed in the USA
LVHW051557181020
669092LV00011B/1065